SIMPLE
MEAL SOLUTIONS
for HIGH CHOLESTEROL

This book is dedicated to my parents, my husband, and my son.

Quarto.com

© 2025 Quarto Publishing Group USA Inc.
Text © 2025 Ashley Reaver

First Published in 2025 by Fair Winds Press, an imprint of The Quarto Group,
100 Cummings Center, Suite 265-D, Beverly, MA 01915, USA.
T (978) 282-9590 F (978) 283-2742

Fair Winds Press titles are also available at discount for retail, wholesale, promotional, and bulk purchase. For details, contact the Special Sales Manager by email at specialsales@quarto.com or by mail at The Quarto Group, Attn: Special Sales Manager, 100 Cummings Center, Suite 265-D, Beverly, MA 01915, USA.

29 28 27 26 25   1 2 3 4 5

ISBN: 978-0-7603-9719-0

Digital edition published in 2025
eISBN: 978-0-7603-9724-4

Library of Congress Cataloging-in-Publication Data available.

Design and Page Layout: Megan Jones Design
Photography: WWH Media, LLC, except Mark Kate McKenna Photography on page 157

Printed in China

The information in this book is for educational purposes only. It is not intended to replace the advice of a physician or medical practitioner. Please see your health care provider before beginning any new health program.

SIMPLE MEAL SOLUTIONS
for HIGH CHOLESTEROL

75 Recipes to Lower Cholesterol
and Support a Healthy Heart

Ashley Reaver, RD

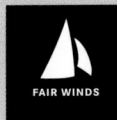

FAIR WINDS

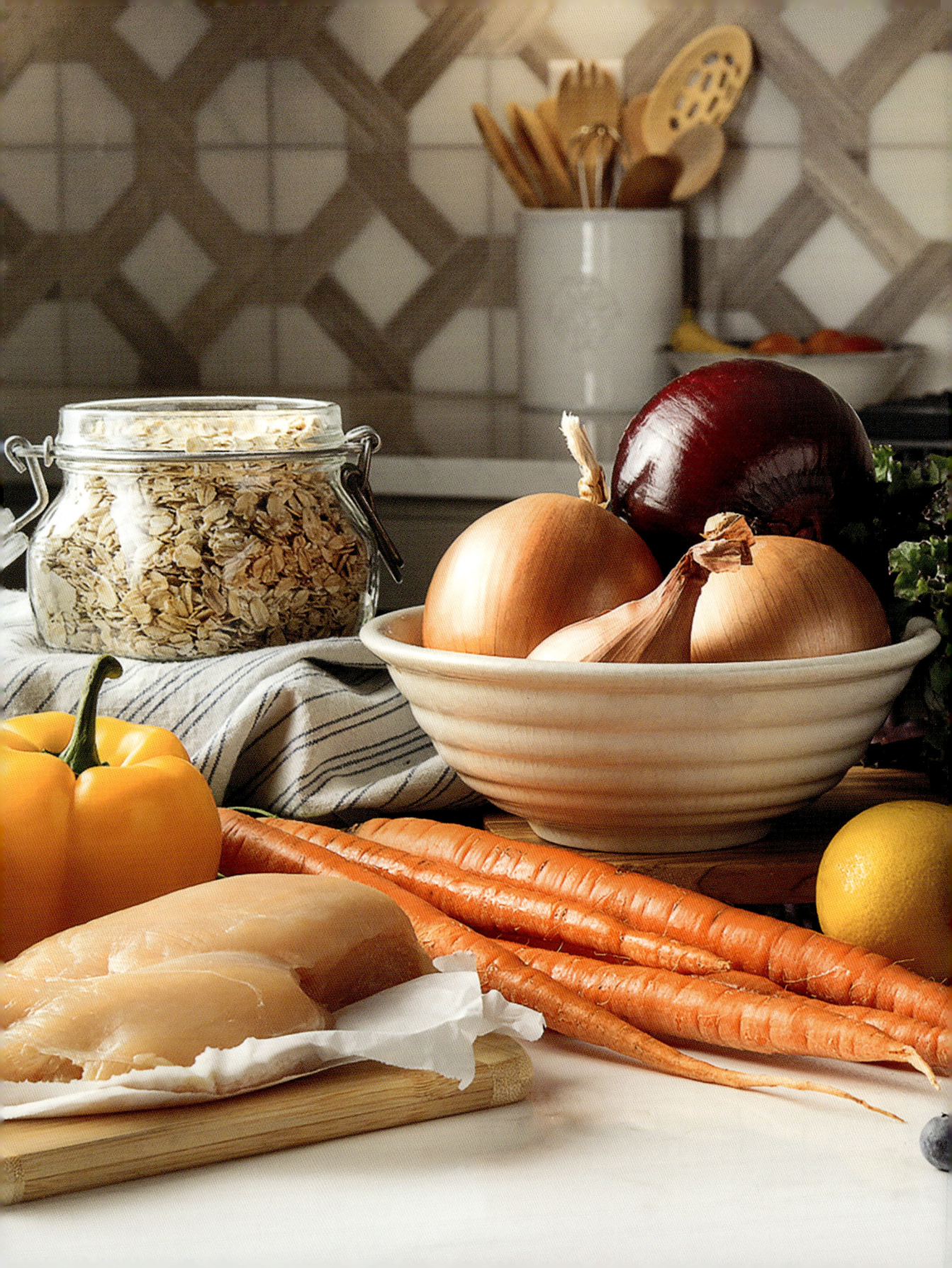

CONTENTS

Introduction

Welcome! Kudos to you for picking up this book and taking your first (or your hundredth) step toward lowering your cholesterol levels. The goal of this cookbook is to empower you to lower your cholesterol with nutrition strategies that target your body's production, usage, and elimination of cholesterol.

If you have found yourself with elevated cholesterol levels, please know that you aren't alone, even though it can sometimes feel isolating. It is estimated that nearly 90 million Americans have elevated cholesterol levels. That is just under one-third of the entire population. It is a very common condition, which explains why statins—the category of pharmaceuticals that target the body's production of cholesterol—hold a few of the top spots on the most prescribed medications list. Fortunately, it's been proven that strategic changes to your diet can lower levels of cholesterol, reduce the likelihood of developing diabetes and high blood pressure, decrease the risk of developing heart disease, and, ultimately, help you live a longer, healthier life. And that's what this book is all about.

Hi, I'm Ashley, and I'm glad you are here! I am a registered dietitian who focuses on helping people lower their cholesterol levels naturally through food and movement. Perhaps like many of you, I have a strong family history of high cholesterol. This inspired me to focus on practical and delicious strategies to not only prevent high cholesterol levels for myself but also serve my family members. I designed this cookbook to be a resource to help you learn about the dietary causes of high cholesterol, identify the best sources of specific nutrients that impact cholesterol, introduce some delicious recipes to your home-cooking repertoire, and help you develop a flexible and enjoyable method for approaching your meals.

One thing you should know about me: I am a serious food lover. You can often find me scanning the grocery store for fun items, checking out new restaurants, and scrolling for recipe inspiration. Growing up in a large, close-knit family that celebrated something together almost every weekend, I spent hours in the kitchen with my mother, aunts, and grandmothers. I know the incredible value of a good meal spent with those you love, which is why I am passionate about not only making heart-healthy food taste delicious but extending the time we have with our loved ones too.

Lowering your cholesterol doesn't have to be painstaking and it doesn't have to mean giving up all the foods you love. In fact, many of the recipes in this book are inspired by family favorites that have been tweaked to be heart-healthier. I hope this cookbook provides meaningful education on the most impactful nutrients for lowering your cholesterol and inspires you to get creative in your own kitchen.

HOW TO USE THIS BOOK

As a nutrition instructor at the University of California, Berkeley, I dedicate the first class of every semester just to reviewing the syllabus. It gives the students the big-picture view of what we will accomplish in the class, provides an overview of what to expect in the course, and highlights how everything ties together over the course of the semester. Since education is a large component of this cookbook, I thought it would be helpful to do a similar "syllabus review."

After working your way through this book, you will have a very clear understanding of the small handful of things you should focus on to lower your cholesterol. You will know the best sources of the most important nutrients for lowering cholesterol. You'll also have 75 recipes that use these ingredients, as well as the nutrition principles taught in the book to help you implement what you've learned.

In today's social media world, anyone with a cell phone can claim to be an expert in basically anything they want. One viral video can undo years of public health campaigns in fewer than 60 seconds. Usually the videos that get the most views are those that contradict mainstream guidance and traditional commonsense advice. This creates a lot of confusion and fear around food choices, which is not helpful when working on long-term solutions for improving your health. Unfortunately, cholesterol and its role in heart disease are not immune to the rampant misinformation available on the Internet. My hope is that this book can counteract some of this noise and help people make better choices for their heart health.

This resource is 100 percent an evidence-based guide on how to lower your cholesterol levels and prevent or delay the development of heart disease. All of the information I present here is supported by scientific research and clinical guidelines. It is important for me to stress that these are proven strategies to lower your cholesterol levels, based on the work of countless researchers, physicians, cardiologists, statisticians, and dietitians who specialize in the field, and demonstrated by hundreds, even thousands, of studies conducted on *humans*. I have taken the research findings and translated them into practical, sustainable, and delicious strategies to lower your cholesterol and decrease your risk of heart disease.

We'll start with a discussion of what cholesterol is, where it comes from, and why it matters in chapter 1. I'll provide an in-depth review of the nutrients that have the most impact on your cholesterol levels and discuss the strategies based on those nutrients that will help you successfully lower them. Chapter 2 walks you through how to prepare for your journey to lower your cholesterol: how to stock your kitchen with heart-healthy foods, time-saving appliances that are worth the investment, and meal preparation strategies to maximize your success. We also discuss how to navigate feeding everyone in your household to reduce battles over food.

The rest of the book is what you came for: recipes that are built specifically for cholesterol management. The recipes are divided into four chapters: breakfast, lunch, dinner, and snacks and treats. Each recipe keeps the most important nutrients for cholesterol management in mind without sacrificing on flavor or requiring hours in the kitchen. Each recipe provides nutrition information to help you track the most important nutrients throughout the day. There are also helpful nutrition or cooking tips included in every recipe to bolster your food knowledge and increase your confidence in the kitchen.

These three components—understanding cholesterol and what impacts it, tools and strategies for success, and delicious recipes to help you implement what you've learned—all come together to help you tackle your cholesterol and improve your heart health. My goal is that you feel confident in knowing that you are doing exactly what you should be doing with your nutrition and can, therefore, ignore all of the other noise and misinformation that will inevitably find its way to you.

No class would be complete without a final exam, right? Consider your regular cholesterol test to be yours. Be sure to get your cholesterol level tested frequently to monitor its progress!

I hope you are feeling that first-day-of-school excitement and motivation. Let's dive in!

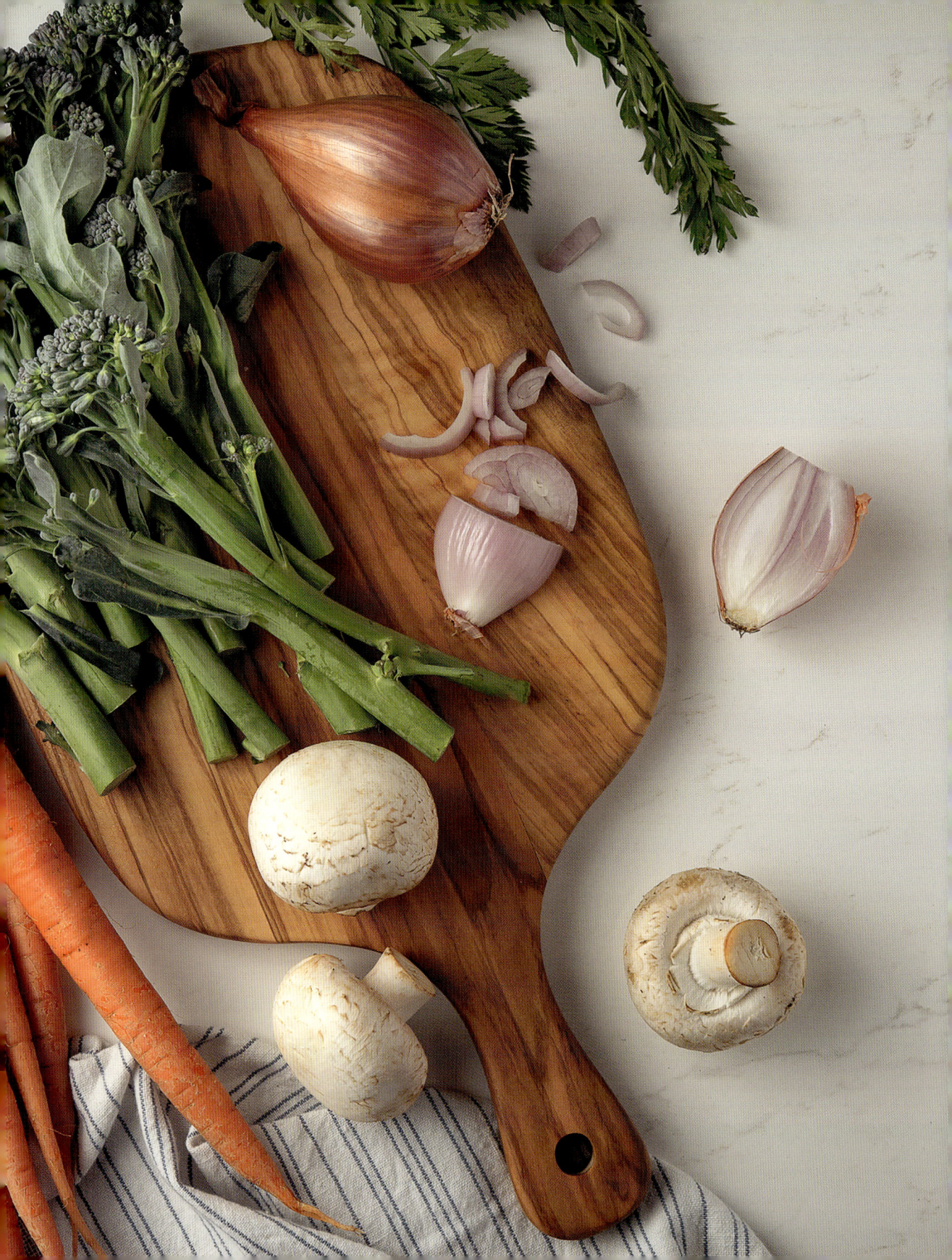

CHAPTER 1

What Is Cholesterol and Why Is It an Issue?

I strongly believe that education is a necessary bridge to action. I don't want you to just blindly follow my recommendations; I want you to understand the "why" behind them. When you hesitate to try a new food, swap an ingredient for a heart-healthier option, or wonder if you really need to eat something this frequently, understanding the specific reasons behind the action will be much more motivating than doing it just "because Ashley said so."

This chapter uncovers the science behind how to lower your cholesterol, hopefully in an approachable and understandable way. Before we can get to the specifics, though, we need to be clear on what cholesterol is, where it comes from, and why it is something we need to worry about in the first place. Only then can you develop a clear understanding of why your nutrition choices can impact your cholesterol level.

Let's start at the beginning.

What Is Cholesterol?

Cholesterol is a waxy fat that is produced by nearly all animals, including humans. It is used for many things in the body: the production of steroid hormones (such as our sex and reproductive hormones), as a building block for cell membranes throughout the body, in the production of bile salts used in digestion, and more. It's important!

Because cholesterol plays so many vital roles in the body, humans are equipped with all of the machinery needed to produce it from any calorie-containing nutrient: protein, carbs, fat, and even alcohol. Contrary to what many people think, roughly 80 percent of our cholesterol is made in the body from these calorie-containing nutrients and only 20 percent comes from our intake of dietary cholesterol. We will come back to this point.

Cholesterol is produced in the liver and usually controlled by a tight feedback loop that shuts off when adequate cholesterol is present in the body. For many people—about one-third of all American adults, according to the Centers for Disease Control and Prevention (CDC)—this feedback loop may become interrupted, resulting in elevated levels of cholesterol becoming present in the bloodstream.

How do we tell when this has happened? Routine blood tests look at *lipoproteins*, which are carriers of cholesterol. Remember, cholesterol is a type of fat, which cannot be transported in the bloodstream on its own. Think of oil and water. When mixed, they will naturally separate after a few seconds, right? Cholesterol works the same way: It must be encased in a fat- and water-friendly package to travel through the blood. The lipoproteins provide that package, and we measure the amount and types of them present in the blood to evaluate cholesterol levels.

Lipoproteins are a combination of proteins and fats that allow cholesterol and triglycerides, the primary form of fat in the body, to be transported through the blood. (For more information on triglycerides, see the sidebar on page 11.) There are four primary types of lipoproteins. Two of them you've likely heard of before: low-density lipoproteins (LDL) and high-density lipoproteins (HDL). The other two, chylomicrons and very-low-density lipoproteins (VLDL), may be new to you, but they are important to understanding the cholesterol synthesis process.

I like to think of the four types of lipoproteins as objects floating in a pool. The more triglyceride (fat) they carry, the lower their density and the better they can float in the water (blood). Here's a quick overview:

- **Chylomicron:** Think of this as a large inflatable unicorn pool floatie. It is primarily fat, with a relatively small amount of protein. After eating a meal that contains fat, our body packages it into a chylomicron so it can be transported around in the blood. Its primary role is to deliver triglycerides to cells in the body to use as energy. Once it has completed its task, a chylomicron becomes a relatively empty vessel (i.e., a chylomicron remnant) and gets transported to the liver and used as the basis to produce other lipoproteins.

- **Very-low-density lipoprotein (VLDL):** Think of this like a beach ball bobbing in the water. It is released from the liver and made using the chylomicron remnant plus additional triglycerides and cholesterol made in the liver. VLDL has a very high percentage of triglycerides, and a relatively small amount of cholesterol and protein. Like the chylomicron, VLDL travels throughout the body distributing triglycerides to be used for energy. Eventually, as the triglycerides it carries become depleted, VLDL becomes an LDL.

- **Low-density lipoprotein (LDL):** LDL is like a soccer ball in the pool. It still floats, but is more compact. It has a low percentage of triglyceride, but a high percentage of cholesterol and some protein. It is considered the primary carrier of cholesterol in the body and delivers it to the tissues.

- **High-density lipoprotein (HDL):** HDL is like a lacrosse ball. Drop one into a pool and it will sink to the bottom. HDL acts differently than the other lipoproteins. Unlike chylomicrons, VLDL, and LDL, which deliver cholesterol throughout the body, HDL is a cholesterol scavenger, picking up excess cholesterol and transporting it back to the liver where it can be degraded or recycled for another purpose. It is primarily protein, with very low amounts of triglycerides and cholesterol. It has other beneficial functions for heart health too, as it has been shown to reduce inflammation in the blood vessels.

The relationship between HDL and LDL is an important one. I like to think of it like cops and robbers. HDLs are the "cops," excess cholesterol is the "robbers," and LDLs are the getaway car. The liver is the jail. But doesn't the liver make cholesterol? Correct! But it also plays a crucial role in removing it from circulation before deciding if it should be repacked as something else needed in the body. Here's how it works: The cops (HDL) travel the streets (our blood vessels) looking for potentially harmful robbers (cholesterol) dropped off by their getaway car (LDL). When HDL finds them, they are picked up and transported to the liver (jail) where they are hopefully rehabilitated into more productive members of society.

A standard lipid panel (the blood test we run to evaluate cholesterol levels) will list the amounts of HDL, LDL, and triglycerides present in the blood. The fourth marker included on the panel is total cholesterol. It's arguably not that interesting,

WHAT ABOUT TRIGLYCERIDES?

Triglycerides are the primary form of fat that we eat and store in our bodies to use as energy. Excess energy from fat, carbohydrates, protein, and alcohol are all stored as triglycerides in our fat tissue. Humans can store a large amount of energy in a relatively small amount of space when using triglycerides. For instance, 1 pound (455 g) of body fat has about 3,500 calories of available energy! While not technically cholesterol, triglycerides still impact heart health. Elevated levels of triglycerides in the blood can indicate too much energy intake, signal other metabolic issues like type 2 diabetes or metabolic syndrome, and overall can increase the risk of developing heart disease. Fortunately, many of the same strategies to lower cholesterol will lower triglycerides too.

though. It is a measurement of the total amount of cholesterol in your body. Total cholesterol can be deceptive: You can have a normal total cholesterol value but a less-than-ideal ratio of HDL to LDL, which is much more important.

WHAT ARE TARGETS FOR HEALTHY CHOLESTEROL LEVELS?

So what is the ideal ratio of HDL to LDL? There are target ranges for cholesterol, but they are dependent on your other risk factors. If we just focus on LDL, the recommendation is "as low as it can go" for most people.

Without any additional risk factors, an LDL of less than 130 mg/dL may be considered acceptable, although the ideal level of LDL is less than 100 mg/dL. If there are other significant risk factors or a previous incidence of heart attack or stroke, an LDL target of 70 mg/dL may be recommended.

Speak with your health care provider to determine the ideal level of LDL cholesterol for you.

There are other measures of cholesterol, and I include more detail on these in the resources section at the end of this book. For the purposes of this book, focusing on LDL is still the most impactful marker, because lowering LDL cholesterol will have the biggest impact on lowering overall cholesterol levels. Plus, the strategies we use to lower LDL will result in the lowering of most other atherogenic cholesterol markers too.

We've covered a lot of information in this section, but here are the key points I want you to take away:

- Cholesterol is transported through the body in lipoproteins.

- LDL is the primary cholesterol transporter in the body.

- A high level of LDL likely means an elevated amount of cholesterol.

- HDL is involved in reverse cholesterol transport, picking cholesterol up from the blood vessels and taking it back to the liver.

Therefore, lower levels of LDL and higher levels of HDL are ideal.

What Causes Elevated Cholesterol?

The easy answer to what causes elevated cholesterol is that your body is making more cholesterol than it needs. As stated in the previous section, cholesterol is produced through a feedback loop in the liver. This feedback loop blocks a crucial step needed for cholesterol production when adequate cholesterol is present. In theory, this should make it nearly impossible for anyone to develop high cholesterol, because the process should halt when there is enough. Unfortunately, it doesn't always work that way.

INTERRUPTING THE FEEDBACK LOOP

The cholesterol production feedback loop can be disrupted in several ways.

Excess Energy Intake

The building block of cholesterol comes from calorie-containing nutrients: carbohydrates, protein, fat, and alcohol. The same processes that convert these nutrients to a form of energy the body can use produce the compound that launches the production of cholesterol. One reason that cholesterol levels can be elevated is if you have too much energy available that results in an excess amount of that compound being present. In other words, consuming more calories than your body requires can lead to high cholesterol.

Insulin Resistance

Another factor that can result in the disruption of the cholesterol-producing feedback loop is having high levels of insulin. Insulin is released when we eat carbohydrates. It is required to move glucose (sugar) into our cells for use as energy. The release of insulin is not a negative or bad thing, but a necessary bodily process. However, if you are *insulin resistant*, your insulin levels are higher following a meal and can remain high even outside of mealtimes—and this can be an issue.

Insulin resistance is a condition that results when our cells don't respond to insulin as effectively as they should. This results in glucose remaining in our bloodstream for longer, potentially causing high blood sugar levels. The body responds by producing more insulin to try to overcome the insulin resistance. This chronically high level of insulin (not the normal spike following a meal with carbohydrates) also pushes past the natural "off" switch on the cholesterol production feedback loop, leading to excess cholesterol production.

Eating within our energy needs and eating and exercising in a way that promotes insulin sensitivity are two key factors for reducing the amount of cholesterol that your body produces. We will come back to these concepts in a bit when we discuss what you can do to lower your levels.

Inadequate Fiber Intake

As we learned in the first part of this book, cholesterol is used in three primary pathways in the body: the production of steroid hormones such as those governing stress and reproduction, as a building block in the outer barrier of our cells, and in the production of bile, a compound that helps with digestion. We don't have very much control over how much cholesterol goes into the production of our stress or sex hormones or in the production of cell membranes. We can, however, influence how much cholesterol is used to produce bile. Spoiler alert: It has to do with dietary fiber intake. If we aren't eating enough fiber, we aren't maximizing the amount of cholesterol we can utilize and, therefore, remove from circulation. The result is higher levels of cholesterol in the blood. More on this later.

Overstaying Its Welcome

The final reason that cholesterol levels can become elevated is simply that cholesterol might be staying in our bloodstream for too long. When our tissues have reached their capacity on how much cholesterol they need to carry out their functions, they stop removing it from circulation.

Think of it as trying to put more water in an already full cup. The cup doesn't increase in size just because there is more water. Similarly, your bodily tissues cannot take in more cholesterol than they need.

One reason that cholesterol may be staying in the bloodstream is that the liver is not removing as much cholesterol as it can. When saturated fat intake is high in the diet, the receptor on the liver that removes LDL may become less effective. With a less effective receptor to remove LDL, more LDL, and therefore more cholesterol, stays in circulation. Low levels of HDL, whose primary role is to pick up excess cholesterol and transport it back to the liver, can have the same effect.

FACTORS *INSIDE* YOUR CONTROL

Dietary Patterns

You've probably realized that many of the causes we've just discussed are influenced by our dietary patterns. The Standard American Diet is how most people eat in the United States. Based on nutrition research and guidelines, it really is not that surprising that many Americans have high cholesterol and, truthfully, I am surprised that it isn't higher! If we consider the causes (high added sugar intake, inadequate fiber, high saturated fat intake, and so on), and how they compare to the Standard American Diet, it doesn't look good. Based on the Dietary Guidelines for Americans, more than 60 percent of adults exceed the recommended intake of added sugars, 90 percent do not meet the recommended intake of dietary fiber, and more than 70 percent exceed the recommended intake of saturated fat. It is hard to estimate calories because they vary based on body size, age, and activity level, but it is likely that Americans are overconsuming calories too, since added sugar is one key factor for excess calorie intake. Additionally, only 25 percent of adults meet the recommended amounts of physical activity that could help to offset additional calorie intake.

Even if you don't follow the Standard American Diet, many popular diets are low in fiber and high in saturated fats. Low-carb diets (like ketogenic, carnivore, Atkins, paleo, and Dukan, to name a few) intentionally restrict whole grains, beans, fruits, and vegetables—where all of the dietary fiber comes from! Even if vegetables and some fruits are included, vegetables are not the best sources of soluble fiber, the most important type of fiber for lowering cholesterol, which you will learn more about later. Furthermore, these diets prioritize protein primarily from animal sources without consideration of saturated fat content. The ketogenic diet takes it one step further and encourages a diet of 80 percent fat, much of which is saturated.

FACTORS *OUTSIDE* YOUR CONTROL

The good news is that there are dietary strategies to try to address the factors we've just discussed—that's the entire point of this book. But there are some things we cannot control. It is worth mentioning them briefly here.

Genetics

Yes, genetics can play a role in elevated cholesterol, but it is often not the most important player. Just like our genetics, we often inherit our eating patterns from our family. What foods we eat often, what foods we never eat, how we celebrate, and how we move our body, for example, are all things we also inherit. If you have siblings or parents who have high cholesterol, it does not necessarily mean that you are genetically doomed and cannot influence your cholesterol. It's important to consider that you all may have a similar dietary pattern that, given similar genetics, may result in elevated levels of cholesterol.

There is a caveat to this: People with familiar hypercholesterolemia, which can be confirmed with a DNA test, have a genetic anomaly in their body's production of cholesterol. For these people,

there is no "off" switch with the feedback loop. No amount of nutrition intervention will impact this. It's important to note that this is not the case with everyone who has high cholesterol. It's estimated that about 10 percent of people with high cholesterol may have one of the two forms of this genetic condition. The other 90 percent—which you most likely fall into—do not have this condition.

Our genetics can influence other ways that our body produces, utilizes, and removes cholesterol, though. This is why families with similar genetics and similar eating patterns may have elevated cholesterol levels, while another family with the same eating pattern but different genetics does not.

Age

Did you know that age is one of the strongest risk factors for elevated cholesterol? This is why most people who have eaten and exercised the same way their entire lives suddenly find themselves with high cholesterol in their forties and fifties. Two things are happening in the body that can help to explain this: We are both making more cholesterol and not removing as much from circulation.

We naturally lose muscle mass as we age. After age thirty, we lose about 10 percent of our muscle mass per decade. By age forty, we have likely noticed a decrease in muscle mass, muscle tone, and muscle strength. Since muscle is our most metabolically active organ, this can result in our body needing less energy. If our calorie intake remains the same, we might find ourselves with extra energy that can go toward cholesterol production. Muscle is also important for insulin sensitivity and, as we know, elevated levels of circulating insulin that can influence our production. Bottom line: Maintaining your muscle mass as you get older is so important for your cholesterol levels.

Our liver also becomes less efficient at removing cholesterol around age forty. This means that less cholesterol is pulled out of circulation.

Naturally, this is going to cause levels of cholesterol, and the lipoproteins that carry it, like LDL, to creep up and potentially fall into that "above normal" range on your next blood test. We can't necessarily influence this, but we can try to offset these changes by supporting healthy cholesterol levels in other ways.

Menopause

For women, seeing a spike in cholesterol levels around perimenopause or age forty-five is likely no surprise. Not only are women dealing with the same loss of muscle mass and decreased efficiency of the liver that happens around age forty as men, but the female body is also drastically reducing its production of sex hormones at the same time. Recall that one of the primary things that cholesterol is used for is the production of sex hormones.

During perimenopause, the roughly five-year period leading up to menopause, hormone production in the ovaries begins to fluctuate and estrogen, testosterone, and progesterone levels begin to decrease pretty dramatically. Menopause is a one-day event that marks the one-year anniversary of a woman's last menstrual cycle. After menopause, levels of estrogen, progesterone, and testosterone remain consistent, although lower than premenopausal levels, with some continued production from the adrenal glands.

While experiencing the fluctuations of hormone production during perimenopause, cholesterol levels can vary widely, and many women will begin to notice increases in cholesterol levels during this time. After menopause, when the majority of the production of these hormones has stopped, women often experience elevated levels of cholesterol.

I'd like to underscore again that these changes to cholesterol levels will likely happen without any change in diet or exercise patterns. Since you are reading this book, you are already taking the steps needed to see how your diet can be tweaked to get those numbers back into the normal range with these age-related changes in mind.

How Does Elevated Cholesterol Impact Your Heart Health?

All of this brings us to why we should care about cholesterol anyway. Simply put, high cholesterol is associated with an increased risk of heart disease. For every 10 percent decrease in your cholesterol levels, you can lower your risk of developing heart disease by 20 percent. That is a pretty amazing return on your investment!

So, what gives? What is cholesterol doing that is so bad for our heart health?

As we learned in the previous section, when the body is producing more cholesterol than it needs, the tissues cannot remove it from circulation at the same rate. This results in cholesterol remaining in circulation for longer, especially LDL. The longer that LDL remains in circulation, the more likely it is to become smaller and denser. These small, dense LDLs are considered particularly atherogenic, meaning that they can lead to the formation of plaques in the arteries.

Small, dense LDLs are more likely to penetrate the walls of the arteries, the blood vessels that carry oxygen-containing blood away from the heart. This can happen in any artery throughout the body and can lead to damage to the arterial walls. This causes the body to mount an inflammatory response, calling in the body's primary defenders—white blood cells—to deal with this damage just like it would in response to any other injury or infection. Small, dense LDLs are also more likely to become oxidized. Once oxidized, LDLs are registered as dangerous foreign invaders that the body tries to protect itself from. This further exacerbates the immune response.

While normally a good thing, our body's immune response to the damage in the arteries and the presence of oxidized LDL does harm. As white blood cells are drawn to the site of the injury in the artery, a specific type of white blood cells, called macrophages, take up the oxidized LDL. Eventually, they die and become known as foam cells. These foam cells accumulate, forming a visible streak on the arteries, termed a fatty streak. Fatty streaks prompt the formation of a fibrous cap to protect it. This is now a plaque, which is a hallmark of atherosclerosis.

Atherosclerosis is the process of accumulating plaque in the arteries, which can lead to the narrowing of these critical vessels that deliver oxygen-containing blood throughout the body, resulting in reduced blood flow. These plaques can also become unstable and break. These breakages result in the formation of a blood clot, which blocks blood flow. When blood flow is completely stopped, it can cause a heart attack or stroke.

Cholesterol plays an absolutely essential role in the development of atherosclerosis, which causes coronary artery disease, the leading type of heart disease in the United States. You cannot develop coronary artery disease without cholesterol, and elevated levels of cholesterol will increase the risk.

OTHER FACTORS CAN ALSO ACCELERATE THE RATE OF ATHEROSCLEROSIS

- High blood pressure: This results in higher amounts of force moving through the arteries to move blood. This can result in damage to the arteries, accelerating the formation of fatty streaks. High blood pressure also increases the risk that there is a breakage of the plaque from the additional force, which can result in a blood clot, leading to a heart attack or stroke.

- Smoking: This habit causes a lot of damage and subsequent inflammation to the lungs. It also introduces many free radicals to the body, compounds that cause oxidation. Smokers are more likely to have oxidized LDL, leading to plaque formation and high blood pressure, increasing the risk of plaque rupture and subsequent heart attack or stroke.

- Diabetes: This condition increases the risk of coronary artery disease through multiple pathways. High levels of blood sugar can independently cause damage to the arteries, increasing the formation of fatty streaks and plaques. It results in elevated levels of insulin, which can increase the production of cholesterol and, therefore, lipoproteins carrying cholesterol, namely LDL. It also can cause stiffening of the arteries, which can increase the risk of developing high blood pressure.

- Other factors: There are other factors like family history of heart disease before age fifty-five for males and before age sixty-five for women, excess visceral body fat in your abdominal cavity, and certain medications. Stress, poor sleep, and even poor dental hygiene can also increase the risk.

What to Do About High Cholesterol

Now that you understand what cholesterol is, how it becomes elevated, and why it's important, let's get into the real reason you are here: what you can do about your high cholesterol. Fortunately, there are strong, research-supported guidelines on how to lower your cholesterol levels. Scientific evidence shows a clear relationship between the dietary intake of specific nutrients and levels of LDL cholesterol, which is why a dietary approach should always be your first option if you have high cholesterol.

This section is the entire basis for this cookbook (I know, I gave you a lot of info before getting here!). All the strategies we're about to discuss should be things you take into consideration when planning and choosing your meals throughout your day. To make it easier, I have built all of the recipes in the cookbook around these strategies. Some recipes are designed to boost your fiber intake, and others are geared toward making some classic recipes a bit lower in saturated fat. Most of them also have more than 20 grams of protein and offer suggestions for how to add more based on your individual protein needs. Don't worry, though: They are just as delicious as they are effective for lowering cholesterol.

So, let's get into it. There are four primary things you can do nutritionally to lower your cholesterol:

1. Eat high-soluble-fiber foods.

2. Limit saturated fat content to less than 6 percent of your overall calories.

3. Eat within your required calorie range.

4. Consume adequate protein to maintain muscle mass.

Let's take these one at a time.

NUTRITIONAL STRATEGY 1: EAT HIGH-SOLUBLE-FIBER FOODS

As we discussed earlier, one of the roles of cholesterol is in the production of bile acids and salts. These are incorporated into bile, a digestive fluid that is made in the liver and stored in the gallbladder. Bile acts as an emulsifier, which allows the fats that we eat to be digested and absorbed.

Typically, bile is recycled at a rate of 97 to 98 percent, so we do not often require new bile production. However, when soluble fiber is consumed with meals that contain fat, the bile gets trapped in the soluble fiber and transported out of the body, since fiber cannot be digested. This requires the body to produce more bile in the liver. It does that by utilizing cholesterol stores.

What Is Soluble Fiber?

There are two primary types of dietary fiber: soluble and insoluble. Soluble fiber dissolves or swells when in contact with water. Insoluble fiber is not impacted by water. A great way to visualize the difference is by thinking of oats and chia seeds versus celery and cucumbers soaking in a glass of water overnight. When you return to the glasses in the morning, the oats and chia will have absorbed much of the water, will have become much softer, and will look very different. On the other hand, the celery and cucumbers will look very similar. The oats and chia are high in soluble fiber, while the celery and cucumbers are primarily insoluble fiber.

SOLUBLE FIBER SOURCES

FIBER SOURCE	SERVING SIZE	SOLUBLE FIBER (g)	TOTAL FIBER (g)
GRAINS			
Barley	½ cup cooked (100 g)	2	6
Brown Rice	½ cup cooked (83 g)	0	2
Oat Bran	½ cup dry (40 g)	2	7
Oats (Instant)	½ cup dry (40 g)	1	3
Oats (Rolled)	½ cup dry (40 g)	2	4
Oats (Steel Cut)	½ cup dry (40 g)	2	4
Quinoa	½ cup cooked (93 g)	1	3
Wheat Bread	1 slice	1	4
FRUITS			
Apples	1 fruit	1	3
Apricots	4 fruits	2	3.5
Avocados	½ medium	2	7
Blackberries	1 cup (145 g)	1	8
Figs, Dried	¼ cup (38 g)	2	4
Grapefruits	1 fruit	2	3
Mangoes	½ fruit	2	3
Oranges	1 fruit	2	3
Peaches	1 fruit	1	2
Pears	1 fruit	1.5	5
Plums	2 fruits	1	2.5
Prunes	3 dried	1	2
Raspberries	1 cup (125 g)	2	4
Strawberries	1 cup (145 g)	1	3

SOLUBLE FIBER SOURCES

FIBER SOURCE	SERVING SIZE	SOLUBLE FIBER (g)	TOTAL FIBER (g)
LEGUMES			
Beans (Kidney, Navy, Black, Pinto)	½ cup cooked (128 g)	2	6.5
Chickpeas	½ cup cooked (128 g)	1.5	4
Lentils	½ cup cooked (99 g)	0.5	5
Lima Beans	½ cup cooked (83 g)	1	4
Peas	½ cup (75 g)	1.5	4
VEGETABLES			
Artichokes	1 cup raw (605 g)	3	10
Asparagus	1 cup raw (125 g)	3	5
Broccoli	1 cup raw (71 g)	2	5
Brussels Sprouts	1 cup raw (88 g)	4	7
Carrots	1 cup raw (130 g)	2.5	4.5
Green Beans	1 cup raw (100 g)	1	3
Okra	1 cup raw (100 g)	2	8
Parsnips	1 cup raw (110 g)	1	7
Sweet Potatoes	1 medium	2	4
Turnips	1 cup raw (150 g)	3.5	10
SEEDS			
Chia Seeds	2 tablespoons (28 g)	2	10
Flaxseeds	2 tablespoons (28 g)	2	8
Sunflower Seeds	¼ cup (36 g)	1	3

Soluble fiber is what plays such a significant role in cholesterol management because it traps the bile after being used for digestion and removes it from the body, hence requiring the body to use more cholesterol to make more bile. Insoluble fiber has many benefits: It helps to fill us up, slows our digestion of foods, and provides excellent "roughage" for normal bowel movements, thereby keeping our colon healthy, but it is not impactful for lowering cholesterol.

We find most soluble fiber in carbohydrate-containing foods, which come from plants. Fiber itself is a carbohydrate, but an indigestible one that humans cannot use for energy. As a whole, most people do not eat enough fiber. The Dietary Guidelines for Americans estimate that 90 percent of Americans do not meet their daily fiber goals—25 grams per day for women and 38 grams per day for men. A focus on eating adequate dietary fiber is a great first place to start when working on your cholesterol levels. Eating a variety of plants—grains, beans, nuts and seeds, fruits, and vegetables—is essential to meeting your daily goal.

An intake of 5 to 10 grams of soluble fiber per day is recommended for lowering cholesterol levels. Unfortunately, soluble fiber is difficult to track because nutrition labels are not required to list the amount of it in a food product. But as long as you're meeting your daily fiber needs while consuming good sources of soluble fiber, you're likely getting enough. The table on the previous page highlights foods that are high in soluble fiber.

NUTRITIONAL STRATEGY 2: LIMIT SATURATED FAT CONTENT TO LESS THAN 6 PERCENT OF YOUR OVERALL CALORIES

Saturated fats have been shown to decrease the sensitivity of the LDL receptor on the liver. As the liver is one of the primary tissues that removes LDL from circulation, limiting saturated fat is critical to maintaining optimal levels of LDL clearance. For most adults, this falls between 10 and 20 grams per day. Unfortunately, more than 70 percent of adults are exceeding the recommended amount.

Suggested intakes of saturated fat per day based on calorie intake:

- 1,500 calories: 10 grams of saturated fat per day
- 1,800 calories: 12 grams of saturated fat per day
- 2,200 calories: 15 grams of saturated fat per day
- 3,000 calories: 20 grams of saturated fat per day

Saturated fats are found in many different types of foods, including both plant and animal products; however, they are typically present in much higher amounts in the latter. Therefore, it follows that monitoring your intake of high-saturated fat animal products will be more fruitful to your cholesterol levels than eliminating your favorite nut. "Healthy" foods like olive oil, avocados, nuts, and seeds do still contain saturated fats, though, so it's smart to be mindful when indulging in them. Refer to the charts on page 23 to see the amount of saturated fats in plant foods and oils.

The chart on page 20 details the amount of total fat, saturated fat, and dietary cholesterol in common animal protein sources. Note that total fat is a combination of saturated and unsaturated fats, which we'll discuss in more detail shortly.

PROTEIN SOURCES			
PER 4-OZ (115 G) SERVING	TOTAL FAT (G)	SATURATED FAT (G)	DIETARY CHOLESTEROL (MG)
MEAT			
Beef, Ground (80/20)	17	8	76
Bison, Ground	8	3	62
Bison Ribeye Steak	3	1	69
Chicken Breast	3	1	82
Chicken Thigh (Skin-on)	19	5	110
Chicken Thigh (Skinless)	5	2	103
Chicken Wing	14	4	124
Eggs (2)	11	4	400
Flank Steak	8	4	56
Lamb Chop	16	7	75
Lamb, Ground	26	11	82
Pork, Ground	20	7	80
Pork Shoulder	20	13	80
Pork Tenderloin	4	1	67
Ribeye Steak	19	9	70
Top Round Roast	4	2	66
Turkey, Ground (93/7)	9	3	92
SEAFOOD			
Cod	1	0	48
Halibut	1	0	55
Salmon	7	1	62
Shrimp	1	0	180
PLANT-BASED			
Beans (Any Kind)	0	0	0
Edamame	6	1	0
Impossible Foods "Beef"	13	6	0
Tofu	3	0	0

What About Dietary Cholesterol?

You'll notice that dietary cholesterol was not mentioned anywhere in our four main strategies for lowering cholesterol levels. Despite years of negative media headlines about eggs, we now know that dietary cholesterol is not as impactful on blood cholesterol levels for most people as we once suspected. In fact, the American Heart Association now recommends that dietary cholesterol intake be kept as low as possible, but no longer recommends that it be limited to less than 300 milligrams per day. This is good news for egg lovers! An excellent source of protein, one or two eggs per day is the current recommendation from the American Heart Association.

This does not mean that dietary cholesterol has no impact at all, but it is not something that should cause you to remove otherwise healthy foods from your diet. Dietary cholesterol is only found in animal products, which is also where we find significant sources of saturated fats, so it's still a good practice to limit them. I recommend one serving of meat from a land animal (chicken, beef, pork, lamb, and so on) per day if you choose to include them.

A surprising fact is that most animal meats, including fish, have roughly the same amount of cholesterol per serving. Refer to the previous chart to see how much dietary cholesterol is found in these common foods.

What about dairy? This deserves a mention, as it is an incredibly common question. The answer is: You do not need to eliminate dairy from your diet to lower cholesterol. Just be mindful of its saturated fat content and choose nonfat or low-fat dairy as much as possible. Dairy products do contain dietary cholesterol, but, as we've just discussed, that's not a reason to cut them out. Plus, it's a great source of nonmeat protein, if you enjoy it.

NUTRITION LABELS

One of the most common questions that I am asked is how to navigate a nutrition label. The things you want to pay attention to when lowering cholesterol are:

- Total fat
- Saturated fat
- Trans fat
- Cholesterol

Unfortunately, the Food and Drug Administration (FDA) does not require monounsaturated fats and polyunsaturated fats to be listed on nutrition labels. This is why the total fat category does not always equal the sum of saturated fat and trans fat: The rest fall into the categories of MUFAs and PUFAs and are not required to appear. MUFAs and PUFAs are the kinds of fats you want to prioritize, however, so you don't need to worry too much about how much of them you're eating as long as you're keeping your saturated fat intake low.

All nutrition labels should have 0 grams of trans fat listed. The use of trans fat was outlawed in the U.S. food system due to its exceptionally negative impact on heart health. Foods must contain less than 0.49 grams per serving, which can be listed as 0 grams. Check nutrition labels for "partially hydrogenated oils," which are trans fats, but may be included in amounts less than 0.49 grams per serving. Avoid trans fats as much as possible.

As we have discussed before, dietary cholesterol is not a nutrient that requires intense focus, and you should not avoid foods solely based on their cholesterol content.

Nutrition Facts

8 servings per container
Serving size   2/3 cup (55g)

Amount per serving
Calories   230

	% Daily Value*
Total Fat 8g	**10%**
Saturated Fat 1g	**5%**
Trans Fat 0g	
Cholesterol 0mg	**0%**
Sodium 160mg	**7%**
Total Carbohydrate 37g	**13%**
Dietary Fiber 4g	**14%**
Total Sugars 12g	
Includes 10g Added Sugars	**20%**
Protein 3g	
Vitamin D 2mcg	10%
Calcium 260mg	20%
Iron 8mg	45%
Potassium 235mg	6%

* The % Daily Value (DV) tells you how much a nutrient in a serving of food contributes to a daily diet. 2,000 calories a day is used for general nutrition advice.

Cheese, butter, and coffee creamers can cause your saturated fat level to creep up each day, so consider some easy swaps: Use cheese as a garnish and not the main event, swap butter for olive or avocado oil, and choose a coffee creamer with no saturated fat. These changes alone could bring your saturated fat content down by 10 grams per day!

What Types of Fats Should We Prioritize?

Unsaturated fats are ideal and should make up the majority of the fats in your diet. There are two different types of unsaturated fats: monounsaturated (MUFA) and polyunsaturated (PUFA). Consumption of MUFA and PUFA, especially when eaten in place of saturated fats, is associated with a favorable lipid profile of normal LDL and HDL levels.

Plant foods, particularly plant oils, nuts, and seeds, in addition to seafood, are great sources of unsaturated fats that are also low in saturated fat. Three plant foods are particularly high in saturated fat, though, and should be eaten mindfully: coconut, palm, and cocoa butter. The tables of common nuts and seeds and fats and oils should serve as a reference for their dietary fat and, in the case of nuts and seeds, dietary fiber and protein content.

NUTRITIONAL STRATEGY 3: EAT WITHIN YOUR REQUIRED CALORIE RANGE

We know that the production of cholesterol begins during the metabolism, or breakdown, of calorie-containing foods, and that excess calorie intake translates to excess cholesterol production in the liver. Therefore, cholesterol levels can be elevated during times of consistent excess calorie intake, which usually coincides with increasing body weight. This is why weight loss is often touted as the main cure for lowering cholesterol, but in reality, just eating within the calorie needs for your current body or stopping weight gain even if you remain at a higher body weight would result in a decrease in cholesterol production.

Unfortunately, the focus on just weight loss completely avoids the two most important nutrients for lowering cholesterol: soluble fiber and saturated fat. In fact, most weight-loss diets drastically reduce soluble fiber by reducing all carbohydrate intake, and increase saturated fat by encouraging very high protein intake. Thus, many people that successfully lose weight can find themselves with even higher levels of cholesterol depending on the method they used to get there.

You can lower your cholesterol levels without losing a single pound. Or, if weight loss is a goal, you can focus on calorie intake and achieve both. Just remember that the high intake of soluble fiber and lower intake of saturated fats should be a part of your strategy too.

NUTS AND SEEDS						
PER 1-OZ (28 G) SERVING	**TOTAL FAT (G)**	**SATURATED FAT (G)**	**MUFA (G)**	**PUFA (G)**	**FIBER (G)**	**PROTEIN (G)**
NUTS						
Almonds	14	1	9	4	4	6
Brazil Nuts	19	5	7	7	2	4
Cashew	12	2	7	2	1	5
Hazelnuts	17	1	13	2	3	4
Macadamia Nuts	22	3	16	0	2	2
Pistachios	13	2	7	4	3	6
Peanut Butter	16	3	8	4	2	7
Pecans	20	2	12	6	3	3
Walnuts	19	2	3	13	2	4
SEEDS						
Chia Seeds	9	1	1	7	10	5
Flaxseeds	12	1	2	8	8	5
Hemp Seeds	15	1	2	12	1	9
Pumpkin Seeds	13	2	5	6	2	2
Sesame Seeds	14	2	5	6	4	5
Sunflower Seeds	16	2	3	11	3	5

FATS AND OILS				
PER 1 TABLESPOON (15 ML)	**TOTAL FAT (G)**	**SATURATED FAT (G)**	**MUFA (G)**	**PUFA (G)**
Avocado Oil	14	2	10	2
Butter	12	7	3	0
Canola Oil	14	1	9	4
Cocoa Butter	14	8	5	0
Coconut Oil	14	11	1	0
Lard	13	5	6	1
Olive Oil (Extra Virgin)	14	2	10	1
Palm Oil	14	7	5	1
Shortening*	13	3	5	4

Contains 2.5 g trans fats, which should be avoided as much as possible.

Exercise Is a Key Component to Managing Energy Intake

Exercise, specifically cardiovascular exercise that slightly increases your heart rate and keeps it elevated, is another great tool for remaining within your calorie needs each day. Walking is one of the best tools we have for increasing energy expenditure. Fitting in as many opportunities as you can to walk throughout the day will result in your body utilizing extra energy that will then not be used toward cholesterol production.

Walking can be in short 5- to 10-minute bursts a few times a day, two 30-minute walks, or one long stroll. Any amount of walking is beneficial to increase your total daily energy expenditure. Exercise comes with many other benefits for heart health too. We will discuss these more at the end of the chapter.

What About Sugar?

Added sugar is a primary factor in the overconsumption of calories. The recommended intake of added sugar is less than 20 grams per day for adults, but more than 60 percent of American adults eat more than that. It's important to stress that "added sugar" does not refer to the sugar that is naturally found in fruits, vegetables, and dairy. This is solely sugar that is added to food products during processing—usually to make it more palatable.

In addition to adding calories, too much added sugar can also increase the risk of developing insulin resistance. Being mindful of added sugar, especially when sedentary, is very important to keep your insulin levels within the normal range. If you have a high-sugar food item, going for a brisk 10-minute walk is an excellent way to help your body manage the rise in blood glucose. This doesn't mean you can never have a sweet treat, but pay attention to when you have them and how frequently.

NUTRITIONAL STRATEGY 4: CONSUME ADEQUATE PROTEIN TO MAINTAIN MUSCLE MASS

Muscle is one of the most metabolically active tissues in the body, meaning that it uses a large amount of energy. An individual with more muscle mass will naturally use more energy. If the body is using more energy, then there will be less excess energy that can be used to create cholesterol.

What is adequate protein? It is calculated based on your body weight, physical activity, and general health goals. A minimum amount of protein that adults should consume to avoid deficiency is 0.8 grams of protein per kilogram of body weight. To calculate this, first determine your body weight in kilograms by dividing your weight in pounds by 2.2. Then, multiply your weight in kilograms by 0.8. For example, a 150-pound person's weight divided by 2.2 gives us 68.18 kilograms. Multiplied by 0.8, this gives you 55 grams of protein per day.

I recommend 1 to 1.2 grams of protein per kilogram of body weight per day for all adults to cover the body's basic needs and support muscle mass while lowering cholesterol. If you are active or are actively trying to lose weight via a calorie deficit, your protein needs may increase to 1.6 grams of protein per kilogram of body weight. For our sample 150-pound (68 kg) person, that is 109 grams of protein per day.

When we consume enough protein, in addition to engaging in moderate physical activity, we increase the amount of muscle we have and the muscles also become more efficient at using fuel, especially glucose. This in turn will help to make us more insulin sensitive, reducing the amount of circulating insulin that may be driving up our cholesterol production. For more on this, see page 26.

It is also important to note that protein can come from both animal and plant sources. An emphasis on plant-based proteins can make it easier to consume more fiber, less saturated fat, and fewer calories, all while providing protein. Soy protein, specifically in minimally processed soy foods like soy milk, edamame, tofu, and tempeh, is independently associated with a reduced risk of heart disease. Swapping out at least one animal protein each week for a plant-based one is an easy way to accomplish all four of the nutrition goals for lowering cholesterol.

BONUS NUTRITIONAL STRATEGY: EAT FRUITS AND VEGETABLES

This is a bonus strategy, but an important one! You probably noticed many fruits and vegetables in the table of good sources of soluble fiber (page 18). You can find soluble fiber in other foods like beans, grains, and seeds, but what you can't get from these foods are antioxidants.

Antioxidants are compounds that help to prevent oxidation. We encounter oxidation often—it's what causes iron to rust, as well as some fruits and vegetables to brown. In our body, antioxidants help to prevent the harmful substances that cause oxidation, *oxidants* or *free radicals*, from causing damage to our cells. When it comes to cholesterol, a diet high in antioxidants can prevent the oxidation of the small, dense LDL particles that makes them particularly dangerous. In other words, while antioxidants won't affect your production of cholesterol, they can help to prevent the cholesterol from becoming especially dangerous.

There are a few antioxidants that deserve your attention every day to protect your heart health: vitamin A (in the form of beta-carotene), vitamin C, vitamin E, and selenium. Be intentional about getting one item from each of these groups a day (see list below). Include a mixture of cooked and raw fruits and vegetables because vitamin C content decreases with cooking, while some forms of vitamin A increase their absorption after cooking.

Here's where you can find these important antioxidants:

- **Vitamin A (in the form of beta-carotene from plants):** This is found in red, yellow, and orange fruits and vegetables, as well as dark leafy greens. The best sources are mangoes, sweet potatoes, red grapefruit, carrots, peaches, kale, and spinach.

- **Vitamin C:** This is found in fresh, frozen, and minimally cooked fruits and vegetables. The best sources are citrus fruits, kiwi, Brussels sprouts, broccoli, bell peppers, and berries.

- **Vitamin E:** This fat-soluble vitamin is typically found in nuts, seeds, and oils. The best sources are sunflower seeds, sunflower seed butter, wheat germ, and wheat germ oil.

- **Selenium:** This is found in Brazil nuts, seafood, meat, poultry, and organ meats. I recommend a daily Brazil nut to help meet your needs!

What Else Can You Do to Prevent Heart Disease?

Elevated cholesterol is just one of the controllable risk factors that influence the development of heart disease. Lowering your cholesterol is a great first step, but you can also work on managing other modifiable risk factors too. Fortunately, eating in a way that lowers cholesterol levels also affects some of these factors, including maintaining a healthy blood pressure, managing blood sugar, and maintaining a healthy weight.

Other steps you can take to reduce your risk factors include:

- Don't smoke, and avoid nicotine exposure.

- Prioritize sleep and aim to consistently get seven to nine hours of sleep each night.

- Engage in the recommended amount of physical activity.

HOW MUCH PHYSICAL ACTIVITY?

The following sections are about physical activity. This is a big one, so it's worth taking some time to talk about it, especially since, as previously discussed, it's good for lowering cholesterol too. There is just no substitution for the benefits of movement on your overall health, but especially your heart health. It is recommended that adults engage in 150 minutes of moderate intensity exercise or 75 minutes of vigorous exercise **and** two sessions of strength training each week. These practices can help to lower your cholesterol and triglyceride levels by increasing your energy expenditure and increasing or maintaining muscle mass. It will also help to increase your insulin sensitivity, which will lower insulin levels, potentially impacting your cholesterol production. Unfortunately, only 25 percent of adults meet the recommended amounts of activity.

"Moderate intensity" or "vigorous intensity" exercise is referring to cardiovascular exercise. We define the intensity of exercise by how elevated your heart rate becomes. For moderate intensity exercise, your heart rate should be elevated, but still in a comfortable range. This is typically 50 to 70 percent of your maximum heart rate. You'll notice that you are breathing heavier, but you'll be able to carry on a conversation at this pace. Vigorous intensity exercise, on the other hand, means your heart rate is running much higher, at 70 to 85 percent of your maximum heart rate. Your breathing will be much heavier, and it will be very difficult to carry on a conversation continuously at this pace. Your maximum heart rate can be calculated by subtracting your age from 220. For example, a fifty-year-old has a maximum heart rate of 170 (220 minus 50), while their moderate intensity range is between 85 and 120 beats per minute.

Cardiovascular activity does so many great things for the body. One of my favorites is that it physically makes our heart muscle larger, stronger, and more efficient! This can decrease blood pressure and our resting heart rate. It also helps to expend extra energy that could otherwise go toward cholesterol production, improves your mood, reduces stress, builds endurance, strengthens the muscles, and makes the muscles more efficient at using fuel (that insulin sensitivity piece again).

But cardiovascular exercise is only one-half of the equation. Strength-training sessions are also vital for building and maintaining muscle mass. Our muscles respond to the stimulus of resistance training by building new and stronger muscle fibers. Couple this with adequate protein intake, and you will have a winning strategy for building muscle mass.

So, what does 150 minutes of moderate intensity exercise or 75 minutes of vigorous exercise plus two sessions of strength training look like in a given week? Some examples include:

- 30 minutes of walking every day and two 20-minute strength-training sessions per week

- Three 30-minute runs and two power yoga or Pilates classes per week

- Two 75-minute bike rides and two 30-minute sessions of gardening

- 2½-hour weekend hike and two 30-minute circuit-training workouts

- Any combination of the above!

Remember, the "best" form of exercise is the one that you do consistently. There is no wrong way to meet these guidelines. Find what you enjoy, and what you can stick with. That will look different for everyone.

Wow, we've covered *a lot* in this chapter! You now understand why we make cholesterol, what influences how much we make, and what causes its levels to be high. We also covered the four nutritional strategies that can directly help you lower your cholesterol level. Then we took a step back and acknowledged that, while critical, cholesterol is just one piece of the puzzle related to your heart health. It is all important to be your healthiest self. I hope that you feel incredibly confident and empowered in knowing exactly what to do in your cholesterol-lowering journey.

Now that you've got all of the knowledge, let's get you set up for success with some practical prep work for implementing the four nutrition strategies.

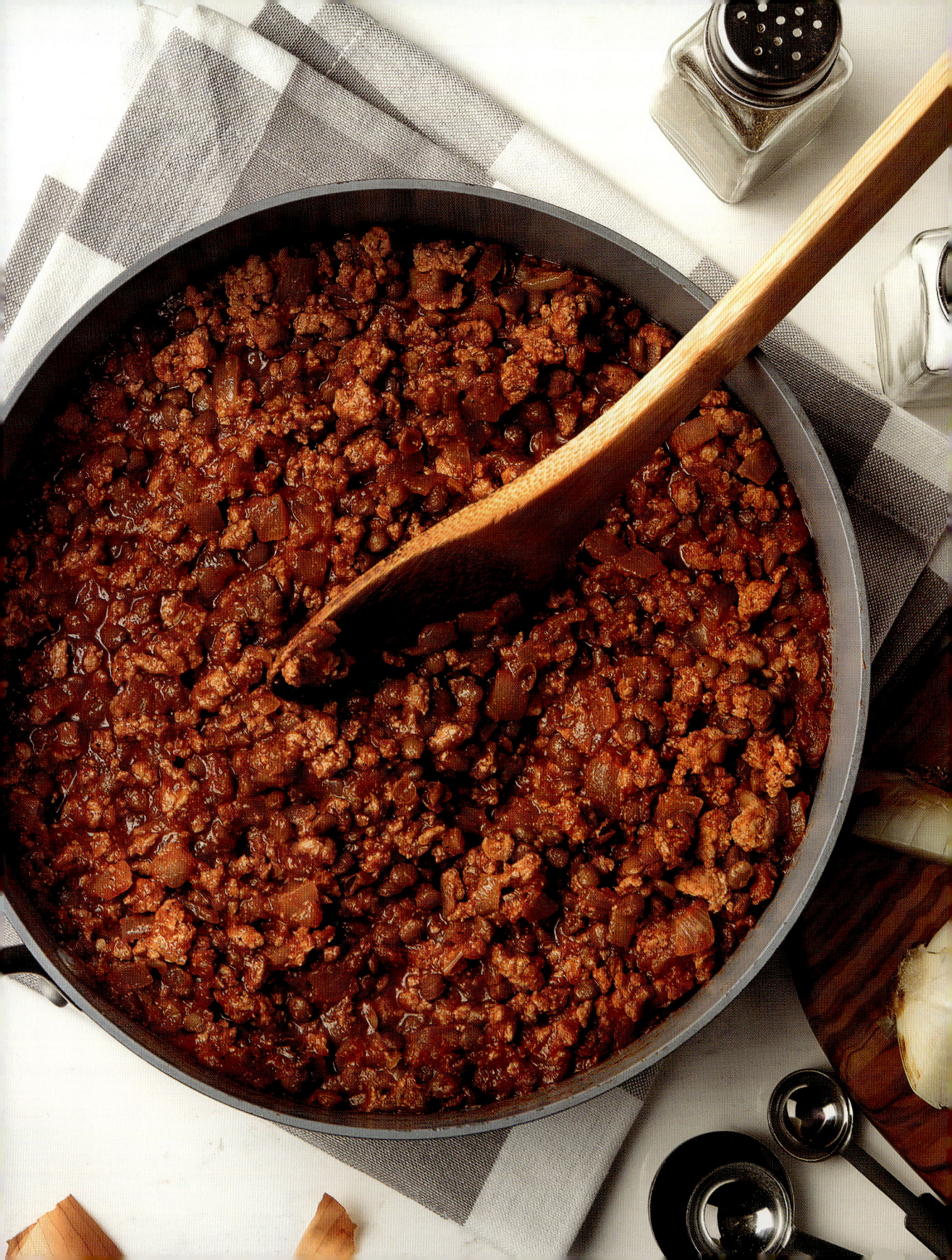

CHAPTER 2

Preparing for Your Lower-Cholesterol Journey

This chapter is possibly the most important one in the book. Of course I want you to understand the nutritional strategies you should be using to lower your cholesterol, but I also want you to be successful implementing those strategies. You can have the best information in the world, but if you can't use it consistently, your cholesterol levels are going to stay the same.

In this chapter, we'll focus on how to do just that. You know now that the backbone of lowering your cholesterol through nutrition is eating enough soluble fiber, monitoring your saturated fat intake, eating within your caloric range, consuming enough protein, and (bonus!) incorporating antioxidants from fruits and vegetables. And while it sounds like a lot to juggle, it is absolutely possible when you have the right tools, ingredients, and strategies.

In this chapter, we'll cover what to keep in your pantry, refrigerator, and freezer to make simple, yet delicious, lower-cholesterol meals. When you have most of these ingredients on hand, it is easy to find suitable options for most of your meals so you're less reliant on takeout. Next up, we'll cover essential kitchen tools and gadgets, including my favorite small appliances that really are worth the investment when it comes to make cooking easier. Then, we'll dive into meal planning and meal prepping. After all, having the food and the equipment doesn't mean that the cholesterol-lowering meals will get made. Just a few simple strategies will save you so much time and mental energy throughout the week. Lastly, we tackle how to navigate other preferences in your household if others aren't on board with your new eating habits. Social support is an incredibly important piece to changing any type of habit, so it deserves its own discussion.

Let's start with the good stuff: what foods to stock!

Stocking Your Cholesterol-Lowering Pantry and Fridge

Prepping your kitchen to support your cholesterol-lowering efforts starts with the food you buy. While this will obviously change some from week to week, having a well-stocked pantry, fridge, and freezer full of heart-healthy staples is incredibly useful when trying to remain consistent in your efforts to improve cholesterol.

The ingredients listed below are my recommendations for stocking a cholesterol-friendly, heart-healthy kitchen. Many of these appear frequently in the recipes in this book and can also be used for those days when you don't have time or can't make it to the grocery store and need to improvise. Pantry staples can be a lifesaver for those times, and it's cost-effective to stock up!

PANTRY STAPLES		
CANNED OR JARRED ITEMS The Stars of Many Meals	**DRIED GOODS** Think High-Soluble Fiber!	**OILS, SPICES, SEASONINGS** Help Avoid Taste Fatigue
Artichoke Hearts	Barley, Pearled	Avocado Oil
Black Beans	Bean-Based Pastas	Chili Powder
Chicken Broth	Brown Rice	Cinnamon, Ground
Chickpeas	Cacao Powder	Coconut Aminos
Kidney Beans	Chia Seeds	Cumin, Ground
Marinara Sauce	Flaxseed, Ground	Garlic Powder
Navy Beans	Hemp Seeds	Italian Seasoning
Pesto	Lentils	Lemon and Lime Juice
Tomato Paste	Nut Butter	Olive Oil
Tomatoes, Diced	Oats, Rolled	Onion Powder
	Protein Powder*	Sesame Oil
	Quinoa	Soy Sauce
	Ramen Noodles	Thyme, Dried
	White Rice	Vanilla

*Protein powder scoops come in all different sizes. Some use two scoops per serving, and some are just one. Plant-based powders tend to require more powder than dairy-based. For all recipes in this book, you want to add 10 grams of protein—not 10 grams of protein powder. Each brand will be different.

FRESH FOOD, FRIDGE, AND FREEZER STAPLES		
FRESH VEGETABLES Long-Lasting Veggies That Add Flavor and Fiber	**FRIDGE STAPLES** Protein Options That Keep for Weeks in the Fridge	**FREEZER STAPLES** More Protein Options and Lots of Antioxidants
Cabbage, Shredded	Eggs or Egg Whites	Berries
Carrots	Low-Fat Cottage Cheese	Broccoli
Celery	Low-Fat Greek Yogurt	Cod
Garlic*	Tofu	Corn
Green Onions		Edamame
Onion*		Mangoes
Salad Blends, Bagged		Peas and Carrots Mix
Sweet Potatoes*		Pepper and Onion Mix
White Potatoes*		Salmon
		Shrimp
		Spinach

Do not refrigerate.

Now that you've got your shopping list, let's talk about the hardware you need to turn those ingredients into delicious meals.

Kitchen Tools and Appliances

You can't cook cholesterol-lowering meals (or any meals for that matter) without the right tools and appliances. This is especially true for the recipes in this book, because the goal is to save you time while lowering your cholesterol. Here's what I recommend having on hand to start making delicious heart-healthy meals.

BASIC KITCHEN TOOLS

- **Glass food storage containers:** The utility of storage containers cannot be overstated. Whether you are preparing ingredients in advance, making recipes in bulk, or storing leftovers for another meal, glass storage containers are a must. Pick up a box with different sizes for different uses.

- **A sharp chef's knife:** Cutting vegetables with a dull blade or one that isn't built for the job will take more time, require more effort, and result in a less consistent product. Invest in a good knife; you will be using it a lot!

- **Cutting board:** After you've got a sharp knife, you'll need a place to use it. While you could get away with one cutting board, I like having two: one for raw meats and seafood and one for fruits, vegetables, and ready-to-eat foods.

- **Mixing bowl:** A large mixing bowl is helpful when putting together ingredients, especially for the recipes in the lunch section. If you only get one, opt for a large one, because it's better to have too much space than not enough.

- **Can opener:** You'll need something to help you open that long list of canned ingredients listed in pantry staples.

- **Meat thermometer:** If you plan to cook animal proteins, you should make sure that you prepare them safely. Even as an experienced cook, I always take the temperature of meats, especially chicken, to ensure I won't experience any negative consequences of undercooked meat.

- **Measuring cups and spoons:** A set of measuring cups and spoons will ensure your recipes come out correctly. If you are a beginner home cook, they will also help you become comfortable with the measurements to be able to "eyeball it" one day.

- **Spatula, rubber scraper, wooden spoon, and whisk:** There are a ton of cooking utensils out there (believe me, my utensil drawer is overflowing), but I think you could accomplish most jobs with these tools.

- **Kitchen shears (or scissors):** You need a good pair. Whether it's opening packages and cutting off bands, trimming meat, or cutting pizza, kitchen shears are multifunctional and make it easier to navigate situations without the threat

of a knife. They can also be used as a vegetable peeler—just use the blade as a knife on potatoes or carrots.

- **Other tools:** A baking sheet, 9 × 13-inch (23 × 33 cm) baking dish, large skillet, and medium pot will cover the majority of all other cooking needs in your kitchen!

KITCHEN APPLIANCES: MY TOP THREE MUST-HAVES TO SAVE YOU TIME

Having a few select appliances in your kitchen can make achieving simple meals even easier. While you can absolutely achieve lower cholesterol levels without these tools, they will help you get cholesterol-friendly meals on the table with much less time and effort. Plus, they help with multitasking!

My top three kitchen appliances for simplifying mealtimes are an electric pressure cooker (I have an Instant Pot), an air fryer, and a high-powered blender or food processor.

Electric Pressure Cooker a.k.a. Instant Pot

The electric pressure cooker, most commonly known as an Instant Pot, is a game changer for weeknight meals and meal prepping! It's basically a pressure cooker with a safety valve, which prevents the scary potential pressure cooker explosions of our grandparents' days. It works by building pressure inside the pot; as the pressure increases, the boiling point of liquids increases too. This means we can achieve higher cooking temperatures than we can on the stove, which translates to faster cooking times. You'll see it used in many of the 30-minute dinner recipes in this book, especially those that would normally take hours to make. Keep in mind that it does take a few extra minutes for the cooker to come to pressure, but this is hands-off time. It also is great for cooking grains, quickly making soups, and even making homemade yogurt.

Air Fryer

The air fryer speeds up cooking times and adds a satisfying and crispy texture to the foods cooked inside of it. Using convection cooking, the air fryer circulates hot air so that foods are constantly in contact with the heat, as opposed to just one side like a dish in the oven. If you don't have an air fryer, you can achieve similar results by placing a wire rack on top of a baking sheet in the oven. In fact, many ovens have a convection setting now. The cooking time will be a bit longer, so pay attention to the internal cooking temperatures in the recipes.

Blender or Food Processer

A high-powered blender or food processor can transform many heart-healthy foods into lots of different things in no time. It's a must-have for quick sauces, puddings, spreads, soups, smoothies, and more.

Honorable Mention: Rice Cooker

If an electric pressure cooker isn't in your future, consider a rice cooker (you don't need both because the pressure cooker has a built-in rice cooking function). They are typically very affordable and make preparing whole grains very easy because they shut off when the grain is ready. While cooking, you can prepare the remaining components for your meal. Cooking times in the rice cooker are typically longer than in an electric pressure cooker.

Meal Planning

Let's start this section with the obvious: You are probably doing more in your life than just trying to lower your cholesterol. Fitting in the extra task of not only cooking meals at home but also making them cholesterol-friendly might feel like just one more thing on your ever-expanding to-do list. And you're right. Grocery shopping and cooking a 30-minute dinner at home takes more time and effort than swinging into your favorite takeout spot.

Unfortunately, hitting your fiber goal or consuming adequate protein doesn't just happen on its own. It takes some intention. To help ease the mental burden and work required to lower your cholesterol through nutrition while juggling the rest of your life, some forethought with meal planning and meal prepping goes a long way.

Planning out your meals can feel intimidating, but it does not need to be. Meal planning can be as simple as *even just thinking about what you will eat*. The point is simply to come up with a few ideas and make sure that you have the ingredients to make them. That's it! It can be as basic as that.

Meal planning is good for people on a journey to lower their cholesterol because it helps you be more intentional about incorporating specific nutrients or types of food into your diet. Some questions to ask yourself as you're getting started include:

- Does it look like you have one or two good sources of soluble fiber each day?

- Do you have too many high-saturated fat items on your weekly menu?

CHECK OUT YOUR SALES CIRCULAR

If you want more variety in your menu, I encourage you to look at the grocery store sales circular for inspiration. You'll not only find ways to make healthy eating more affordable, but produce that goes on sale is typically in season, so it is the freshest option. The sales typically change weekly or biweekly, making it a great way to infuse some variety in your menu and inspire you to try out different ingredients.

- Do you have a protein source at each meal?

- Do you have at least two different fruits and three vegetables each day?

If you want to take a more structured approach to meal planning, I recommend a different approach than what you might expect from a registered dietitian: Keep it simple. After working with clients for more than 10 years, I can confidently say that highly structured meal plans don't work. Everyone thinks that they want someone to "just tell me what to eat," but in reality, we all need more flexibility. That's why I focus so much on the knowledge of how to make food decisions anywhere, at any time, that support your cholesterol.

Life happens and things don't always go according to plan. You may run late one night, have an unexpected lunch meeting, or need to grab a quick dinner between your kids' practices. If your meals are strictly planned every day, with no room for life's unexpected obstacles, you aren't likely to be successful, which is very unmotivating for your meal planning the following week.

Instead, I recommend choosing a handful of recipes to cover your meals (outlined on the next page) and purchasing those ingredients with just one trip to the store each week. Lean on your pantry staples when you need to make dinner, but don't have anything specific planned. Having fewer options, embracing leftovers (this is key!), and using your pantry staples will cut down on your work throughout the week, reduce the potential of food waste, and make incorporating cholesterol-friendly meals *consistently* easier. Our goal is to set up sustainable habits, not to burn you out after one month.

My strategy for simple weekly meal planning:

- Choose two breakfast recipes—one sweet and one savory.

- Have two options for lunch—these should be foods you will eat only for lunch. You can include planned dinner leftovers to fill gaps.

- Choose four dinner recipes—these should include a mixture of difficulty ranging from pantry- or freezer-only ingredients to a full 30-minute meal. If possible, try to make extra portions to use the other nights or for lunches.

A SAMPLE OF WHAT THAT COULD LOOK LIKE WITH RECIPES FROM THIS BOOK							
	SUNDAY	MONDAY	TUESDAY	WEDNESDAY	THURSDAY	FRIDAY	SATURDAY
Breakfast	Mocha Chia Seed Pudding (page 42)	Egg Salad (page 46)	Mocha Chia Seed Pudding	Egg Salad	Mocha Chia Seed Pudding	Egg Salad	Mocha Chia Seed Pudding
Lunch	Three-Bean Salad with Edamame (page 63)	Chicken and Barley Stir-Fry (leftovers)	Three-Bean Salad with Edamame	Tofu Taco Salad (leftovers)	Weeknight Beef Stew (leftovers)	Lemony Chicken Soup (page 66)	Lemony Chicken Soup
Dinner	Chicken and Barley Stir-Fry (page 97)	Tofu Tacos (page 103)	Weeknight Beef Stew (page 112)	Out	Air-Fryer Salmon Bites with Cauliflower Stir-Fry (page 132)	Out	Clean out the fridge! Have a meal of any leftovers or ingredients.

Meal Prepping

Whereas meal planning is mostly the mental work of thinking about your meals, their nutrients, and the needed groceries to accomplish them, meal prepping actually involves the manual work of getting some ingredients or meals prepared. Meal prepping does not have to require hours in the kitchen on Sunday to make all of your meals for the week. Setting aside even just one hour each week for preparing some of your ingredients can save you hours over the course of the week. Be strategic and maximize your time in the kitchen.

If you can find the time, I recommend getting these tasks out of the way:

- Cut up all of the vegetables you will need for your recipes. It will make your weeknight dinners come together even faster.

- Cook your grains. These take time to cook, especially barley and brown rice. If you get these out of the way, your dinners may come together even faster.

- Prep breakfast. Breakfast is the easiest meal to overlook. Just like your other meals, though, it won't just happen without some thought.

Some recipes can be made in advance and will taste even better after sitting in the fridge for a day or two. Soups and stews usually fit this bill. While you are in the kitchen prepping veggies, grains, and breakfast, try tossing a meal into the oven or electric pressure cooker to take the work away from another time.

BATCH COOKING

As a time-saving hack, I can't recommend batch cooking enough, especially for things like grains. Batch cooking is making a larger quantity of an ingredient than you need for one meal. It saves time, energy, and effort across your whole week. Here's what batch cooking can look like:

- Tripling the amount of barley, quinoa, or rice required for a recipe. Save some for another dinner during the week. Freeze the rest in silicon molds so they can easily be used for quick lunches or dinners.

- Double the protein you are cooking by adding another sheet pan to the oven while you are already cooking dinner. Use the extra protein for lunches paired with bagged salad blends, frozen grains, or vegetables, or added to canned vegetable soup.

- Depending on your family size, you might not be able to depend on dinner leftovers for lunch. Consider doubling a recipe and using it as your lunch for a day or two during the week.

Explaining Your Cholesterol Journey to Your Family

One thing that can be particularly challenging when making changes to your food routine is getting others on board with the changes too. This is particularly applicable to other members of your immediate household who will notice a change in ingredients and recipes even though they did not make the decision to improve their cholesterol levels.

These are the strategies I've found that work the best for my clients who struggle with this:

EXPLAIN WHAT YOU'RE TRYING TO ACCOMPLISH

First and foremost, explain why you are making the changes. Anyone who loves and cares about you (as your partner and children should) will want you to be around—and healthy—for as long as possible. Be up front with the adults in your household that you are working to lower your cholesterol. Tell the kids that you want to make sure your heart is as healthy as possible, and isn't it really cool that you can do that through the foods that you eat?

INVOLVE EVERYONE IN WEEKLY MEAL PLANNING

Figuring out what to eat for yourself twenty-one times a week is exhausting. Adding on twenty-one meals for each additional person makes it only harder. Still worse is when they complain about what you've made. Involving everyone in meal planning will give each person at least one night that they can be excited about dinner. If they don't like what is being served on the other nights, it's important to remind them that it is not their night to choose dinner and that everyone else also gets a turn. Teaching them that every meal will not be their favorite is a good skill to build. You might say, "But my kids will just pick pizza or chicken tenders every night," and I say that's okay. Are those the best choices for your cholesterol every night? Probably not, but you can add other things to your plate that are more in-line with your nutrition goals. And while you're doing that, why not give your kids a little bit too? Introduce some new foods next to their favorites. That brings us to the last point.

ADD INGREDIENTS THAT REFLECT THE FOUR NUTRITIONAL STRATEGIES

Don't be afraid to add things to your meals that help you increase the fiber content, get in enough protein, add some antioxidants from fruits or vegetables, and be mindful of your saturated fat intake. Here's where meal prepping, batch cooking, and having a stocked pantry and freezer can come in to save the day. You do not need to make a completely separate meal for yourself. In fact, I would say it's better for your family not to see you avoid their favorite foods or tell them that you "can't" eat something. Instead, customize it. Chicken tenders and macaroni and cheese again? Can you add a side of microwaved or steamed broccoli? Pizza can easily be made into a complete meal by adding a bagged salad to the plate with some leftover shredded chicken. Taco night? Add beans to it and cut back on the cheese. You can make these tweaks without needing to spend hours in the kitchen.

You need support when you are trying to make dietary changes for your health. It is already hard. It is even harder when you are met with complaints at every single meal period. You do not need to strive for perfection. Strive for better than your usual. Control what you can and release what you can't. If you have one meal that is not ideal, remember that you have twenty other opportunities to focus on your cholesterol each week. Don't give up!

On that note and without further ado, it's time to roll up our sleeves and dive into the recipes themselves. Each dish in the following chapters was created with simplicity, taste, and your cholesterol in mind. They incorporate the nutrition strategies outlined in chapter 1. Let's get cooking!

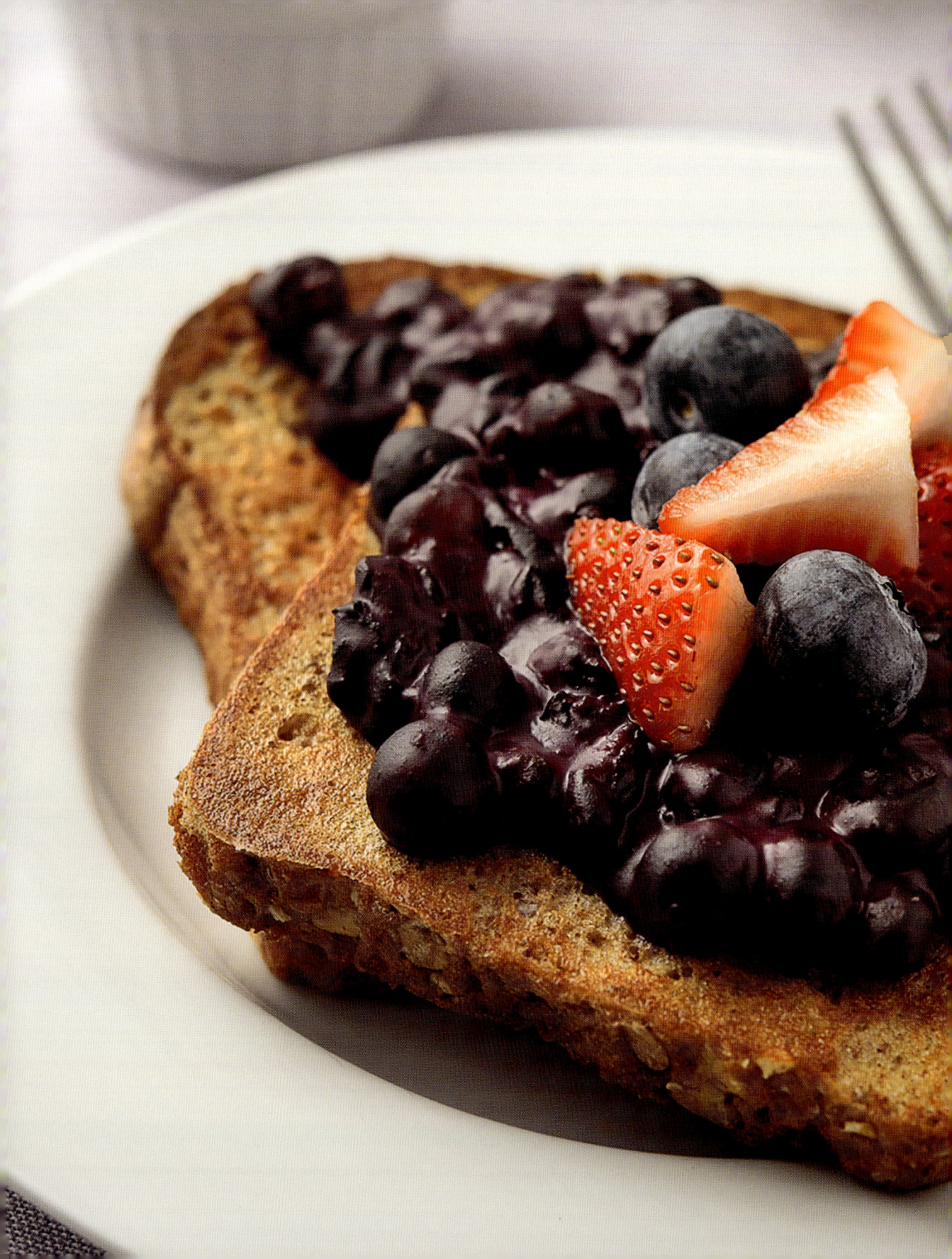

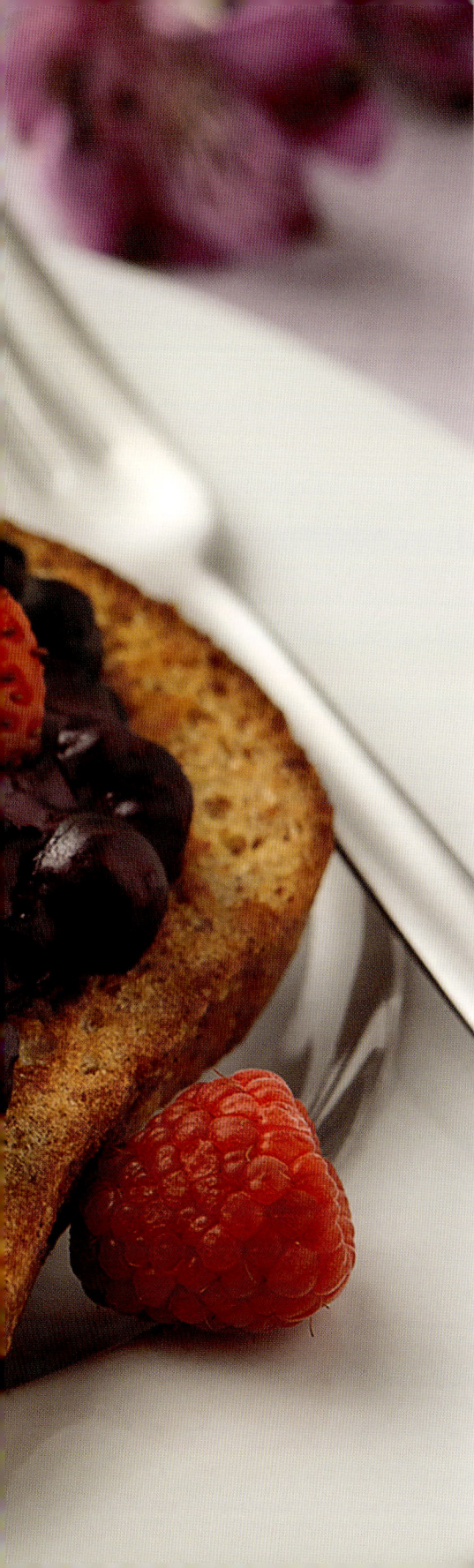

CHAPTER 3

15 Breakfasts in 15 Minutes

In my opinion, breakfast is the biggest opportunity to improve your nutrition. Many people skip it or simply grab a quick bite that does not help them meet their protein or fiber goals. All of the breakfast recipes in this chapter contain at least 20 grams of protein and 6 grams of fiber. This will not only help you tackle your goals for the day but keep you satisfied until lunch time. Enjoy!

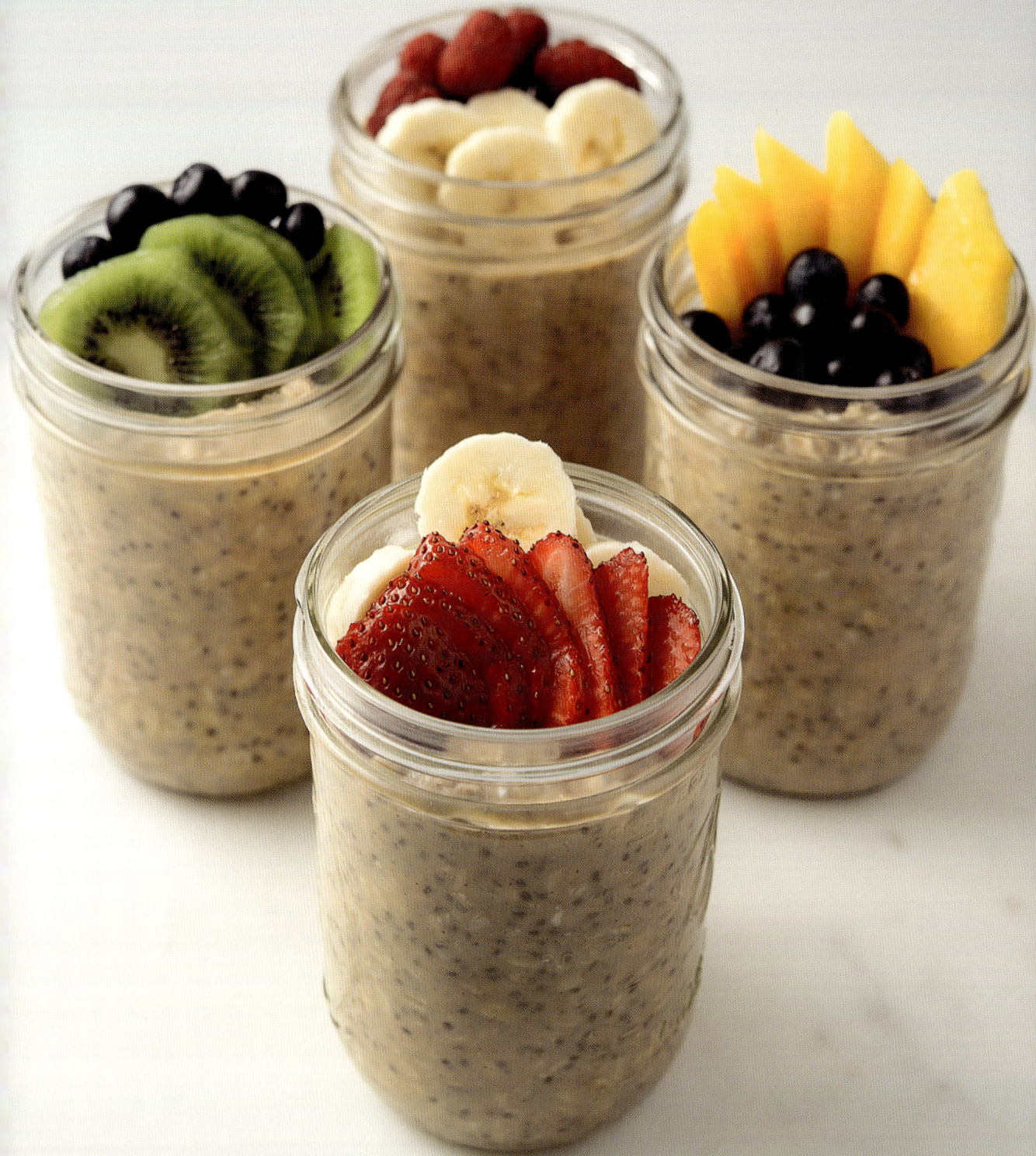

EVERYDAY OVERNIGHT OATS

■ **YIELD:**
1 SERVING

■ **PREP TIME:**
5 MINUTES

■ **COOK TIME:**
0 MINUTES

Oats are often recommended for lowering cholesterol because they are high in a particular type of soluble fiber, called beta-glucan. This "sticky" soluble fiber is the most effective for binding to bile salts and preventing their reabsorption. This simple recipe is a win-win-win: It can be made in advance for an easy grab-and-go-breakfast; it tastes delicious; and it starts your day with a significant amount of beta-glucan. Use the base recipe and vary the add-ins. The possibilities are endless!

⅔ cup (67 g) rolled oats

1 tablespoon (10 g) chia seeds

¼ teaspoon ground cinnamon

Vanilla protein powder, enough to add 10 g of protein (see Notes)

2 tablespoons (11 g) powdered peanut butter

1 cup (235 ml) soy milk or low-fat milk

Add rolled oats, chia seeds, cinnamon, vanilla protein powder, powdered peanut butter, and soy milk or low-fat milk to a glass container like a mason jar. Stir with a spoon or top with a lid and shake to thoroughly combine. Place the sealed container in the refrigerator overnight to chill.

In the morning, simply remove the lid from your container and add your desired toppings. Alternatively, you can spoon the overnight oats into a bowl and add your toppings there.

SUGGESTED TOPPINGS

Mixed berries

Raspberries

Mango

Kiwi

Banana

Raisins

Diced prunes

Chopped walnuts

Chopped pistachios

Sliced almonds

NOTES

- You can turn this recipe into pumpkin overnight oats by adding ¼ cup (61 g) pureed pumpkin and 1 teaspoon maple syrup, and swapping the cinnamon for pumpkin spice.

- Protein powder scoops come in all different sizes. Some use two scoops per serving, and some are just one. Plant-based powders tend to require more powder than dairy-based.

- For all recipes in this book, you want to add 10 grams of protein—not 10 grams of protein powder. Each brand will be different.

NUTRITIONAL ANALYSIS
(base recipe)

SERVING SIZE: About 1½ cups (about 200 g) overnight oats

PER SERVING: 463 calories; 14 g fat; 1 g saturated fat; 37 g protein; 42 g carbohydrate; 12 g dietary fiber

MOCHA CHIA SEED PUDDING

Looking for breakfast that does double duty as your morning coffee? Look no further! Packed with fiber from the chia seeds, this pudding also gives you a caffeine boost from the instant coffee, making it a perfect grab-and-go breakfast option!

■ **YIELD:**
4 SERVINGS

■ **PREP TIME:**
5 MINUTES

■ **COOK TIME:**
0 MINUTES

1 cup (161 g) chia seeds

Chocolate protein powder, enough to add 10 g of protein

2 tablespoons (14 g) instant coffee

4 cups (946 ml) soy milk

2 tablespoons (15 g) cocoa powder

1½ teaspoons vanilla extract

Add chia seeds, chocolate protein powder, instant coffee, soy milk, cocoa powder, and vanilla extract to a high-power blender or food processor and blend on high for approximately 90 seconds or until mixture is creamy. Alternatively, combine all the ingredients in a large dish, add the dish to the refrigerator to chill overnight, and blend in the morning. This may result in a smoother pudding, depending on the power of your machine.

Mocha Chia Seed Pudding can be enjoyed immediately or stored in the fridge for up to 1 week. The texture will continue to thicken when chilled.

To serve, portion the pudding into 4 individual dishes.

NOTES

- This makes a great dessert too, but don't add the instant coffee if you are planning to enjoy the pudding close to bedtime.

- You can substitute the instant coffee for 1 cup (235 ml) strong black coffee. If you go this route, reduce the soy milk by 1 cup (235 ml).

- The sweetness of this pudding depends on the sweetness of your protein powder. If you'd prefer a sweeter pudding, add 1 teaspoon maple syrup.

NUTRITIONAL ANALYSIS

SERVING SIZE: About 1¼ cups (about 341 g) chia seed pudding

PER SERVING: 427 calories; 24 g fat; 3 g saturated fat; 29 g protein; 30 g carbohydrates; 12 g dietary fiber

BANANA OAT PANCAKES

Want all the benefits of oats without having to eat a bowl of oatmeal? Try these Banana Oat Pancakes. These pancakes are surprisingly light and fluffy, despite having 6 grams of fiber and 9 grams of protein per serving—about three to four times more than a regular pancake. Make a large batch of these on the weekend and reheat them in the microwave or toaster for weekday breakfasts that have a weekend feel.

■ **YIELD:**
2 SERVINGS

■ **PREP TIME:**
5 MINUTES

■ **COOK TIME:**
5 MINUTES

1 cup (80 g) rolled oats

1 ripe banana

1 egg

1 teaspoon baking powder

½ teaspoon vanilla extract

½ teaspoon ground cinnamon

1 teaspoon olive or avocado oil

½ cup (120 ml) + 1 tablespoon (15 ml) skim, low-fat, or soy milk

Nonstick cooking spray

TOPPING OPTIONS

2 tablespoons (32 g) nut or seed butter of choice, such as peanut, almond, or sunflower seed

½ cup (75 g) fresh or frozen and microwaved berries

2 ounces (55 g) turkey sausage or turkey bacon

Add rolled oats, banana, egg, baking powder, vanilla extract, ground cinnamon, olive or avocado oil, and milk to a blender. Blend for about 30 seconds or until all ingredients have combined into a cohesive batter.

Heat a large skillet over medium heat. Spray with nonstick cooking spray. Cook each pancake for 3 to 4 minutes or until you see small bubbles form around the edge of the pancake. Flip and cook for another 3 to 4 minutes. This recipe should make two 8-inch (20 cm) pancakes or four 4-inch (10 cm) pancakes.

Serve with your preferred toppings and enjoy!

NOTES

- What's the difference between baking soda and baking powder? Baking powder contains an acid to activate the bubbles. Baking soda is used in recipes that provide the acid from other ingredients (surprisingly, brown sugar provides the acid in cookie recipes). Since we don't have acidic ingredients in this recipe, baking soda cannot be subbed for baking powder. However, if soda is all you have, adding a small amount of lemon juice (½ teaspoon [3 ml]) to the blender can add enough acid.

- These pancakes also are a great option for a sweeter tortilla-like wrap. If you are a big fan of pigs in a blanket, use one of these pancakes!

- You can also use this batter as a waffle mix. Omit the extra tablespoon (15 ml) of milk.

NUTRITIONAL ANALYSIS

SERVING SIZE: One 8-inch (20 cm) pancake or two 4-inch (10 cm) pancakes

PER SERVING: 329 calories; 8 g fat; 2 g saturated fat; 9 g protein; 45 g carbohydrate; 6 g dietary fiber

PB&J FRENCH TOAST

Good news—you can still eat French toast and lower your cholesterol. A few simple alterations make this French toast friendlier for cholesterol, none of which include cutting out the egg—remember, we don't need to. Use high-fiber bread, swap the syrup for mixed berries, add some additional protein and healthy fats with peanut butter, and you're good to go.

■ **YIELD:**
1 SERVING

■ **PREP TIME:**
5 MINUTES

■ **COOK TIME:**
10 MINUTES

1 whole egg

¼ cup (60 ml) egg whites

⅛ teaspoon ground cinnamon

¼ teaspoon vanilla

2 slices 100 percent whole wheat bread

Nonstick cooking spray

½ cup (75 g) fresh or frozen berries

1 tablespoon (16 g) peanut butter

Whisk the egg and egg whites with cinnamon and vanilla in a medium bowl until smooth. Submerge one of your bread slices in the mixture and allow to soak for 1 to 2 minutes on each side.

Spray a medium sauté pan with nonstick cooking spray and place over medium heat. Add bread to the pan and cook for 3 to 4 minutes on each side or until golden brown. Repeat this process with the second slice.

Add berries to a microwave-safe dish and microwave for 30 seconds, then open the microwave and give the dish a quick stir. Microwave for another 30 more seconds or so until berries are warm and can be easily mashed with a fork. Frozen berries will produce a bit more juice than fresh berries.

Plate your French toast, spread half the peanut butter on top, then pour over half the warmed berries. Serve and enjoy!

NOTES

- Egg whites do not contain any cholesterol or saturated fat. They are essentially 90 percent water and 10 percent protein, making them an excellent way to boost the protein content of meals. If you don't have egg whites, using another whole egg is an option.

- This is a great make-ahead breakfast option. Cook a few servings, store in the refrigerator, and reheat in the toaster before serving.

- Serve with ½ cup (120 ml) of scrambled egg whites on the side to increase the protein content of this meal by 13 g.

NUTRITIONAL ANALYSIS

SERVING SIZE: 2 slices French toast with toppings

PER SERVING: 380 calories; 15 g fat; 3 g saturated fat; 21 g protein; 35 g carbohydrate; 6 g dietary fiber

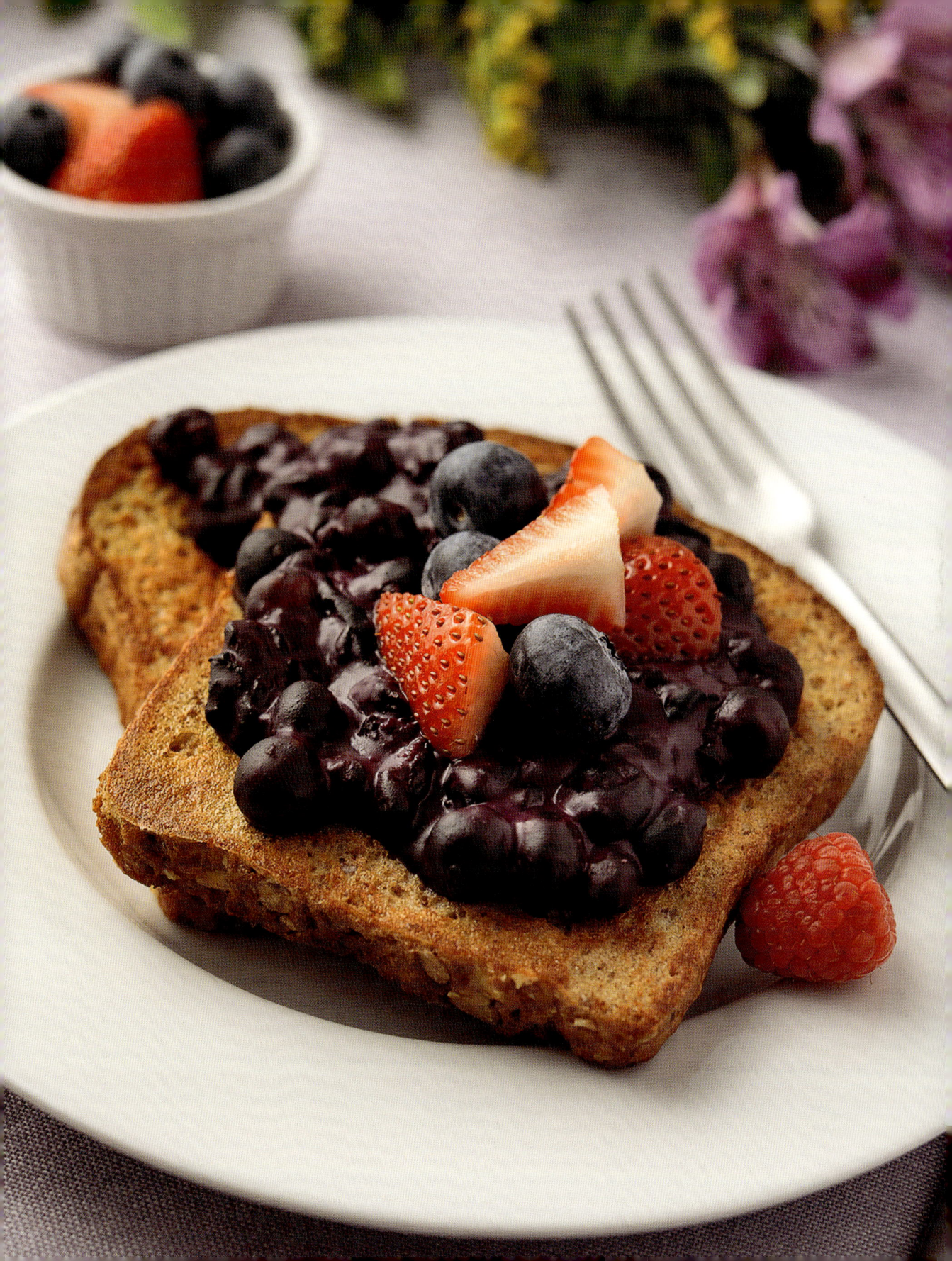

EGG SALAD

■ YIELD:
4 SERVINGS

■ PREP TIME:
5 MINUTES

■ COOK TIME:
10 MINUTES

What?! Egg salad in a book on lowering cholesterol?! Yes! I encourage you to revisit chapter 1 if you're shocked. According to the American Heart Association, most people with high cholesterol can enjoy 1 to 2 eggs per day without negative impacts on their cholesterol levels since dietary cholesterol has minimal impacts on blood cholesterol. Egg salad is an incredibly easy make-ahead breakfast or lunch option. In my version, I remove half of the yolks so they don't overpower the dish, and this cuts down on the saturated fat.

8 eggs

1½ tablespoons (21 g) mayonnaise

1½ teaspoons yellow or spicy brown mustard

1½ teaspoons your favorite everyday seasoning blend (see Note)

2 celery stalks, diced

2 green onions, both green and white parts, sliced

8 slices whole-grain bread, toasted

Lettuce

Tomato

Red onions

Pickles

Add eggs to a medium saucepan and cover with water. Cover with a lid and place on the stove over high heat until the water boils. Remove from heat and allow to sit for 10 to 12 minutes or until the yolks are hard.

Prepare an ice bath by filling a bowl with ice and water. When the eggs are done, pour off hot water and shake eggs in the pan until they crack (this will make them easier to peel). Then submerge the eggs into the ice bath to stop the cooking process. Begin to peel the eggs, placing them back in the cold water once peeled.

Once all of the eggs are peeled, cut the eggs in half and remove the yolks. Add 4 whole yolks to a bowl and mash with a fork. Reserve 4 yolks for another purpose. Add mayonnaise, mustard, seasoning blend, celery, and green onions, and stir until a cohesive mixture forms.

Dice your egg whites, add to the yolk mixture, and stir to combine.

Serve as an open-faced sandwich on top of 2 pieces of toasted high-fiber bread. Top with lettuce, tomato, red onion, pickles, or your other favorite sandwich garnishes.

NOTE

Seasoning blends are usually a mixture of spices that taste good on basically everything. Some well-known ones are Old Bay, Season-All, or Kinder's All Purpose, to name a few. Note that all of these seasonings contain salt. If you use a different seasoning blend, consider that you may need to add salt.

NUTRITIONAL ANALYSIS

SERVING SIZE: 1 sandwich

PER SERVING: 320 calories; 17 g fat; 4 g saturated fat; 20 g protein; 30 g carbohydrate; 7 g dietary fiber

SMOKED SALMON SPREAD

YIELD:
2 SERVINGS

PREP TIME:
5 MINUTES

COOK TIME:
0 MINUTES

If you are a fan of bagels for breakfast, this spread is a great option that will help you increase your protein consumption. Compared with cream cheese, cottage cheese has about 10 grams more protein and 80 percent less fat. Plus, when blended, cottage cheese becomes very creamy and spreadable. The smoked salmon also provides heart-healthy omega-3s.

½ cup (115 g) 2 percent cottage cheese

½ green onion, both green and white parts, roughly chopped

2 ounces (57 g) smoked salmon

2 slices whole wheat bread

Red onion

Capers

Cucumber

Tomato

Everything bagel seasoning

1 cup (145 g) blueberries

Add cottage cheese to a food processor and process on high for 30 to 60 seconds until it is completely creamy with no visible lumps. Next, add green onion and pulse 4 to 5 times to break up. Finally, separate the smoked salmon so it is not stuck together and add to the food processor. Pulse 3 to 4 times until the salmon is broken into small bites but not completely blended into a paste.

Toast your bread. Evenly divide the spread between 2 slices. Top with your favorite bagel toppings like red onion, capers, cucumber, tomato, and everything bagel seasoning.

Serve with ½ cup (72 g) blueberries on the side of each serving, and enjoy!

NUTRITIONAL ANALYSIS

SERVING SIZE: 1 open-face sandwich + ½ cup (72 g) blueberries

PER SERVING: 342 calories; 8 g fat; 3 g saturated fat; 34 g protein; 35 g carbohydrate; 8 g dietary fiber

NOTE

This recipe can be made ahead and stored in the fridge for a few days to mark breakfast off your to-do list for the week.

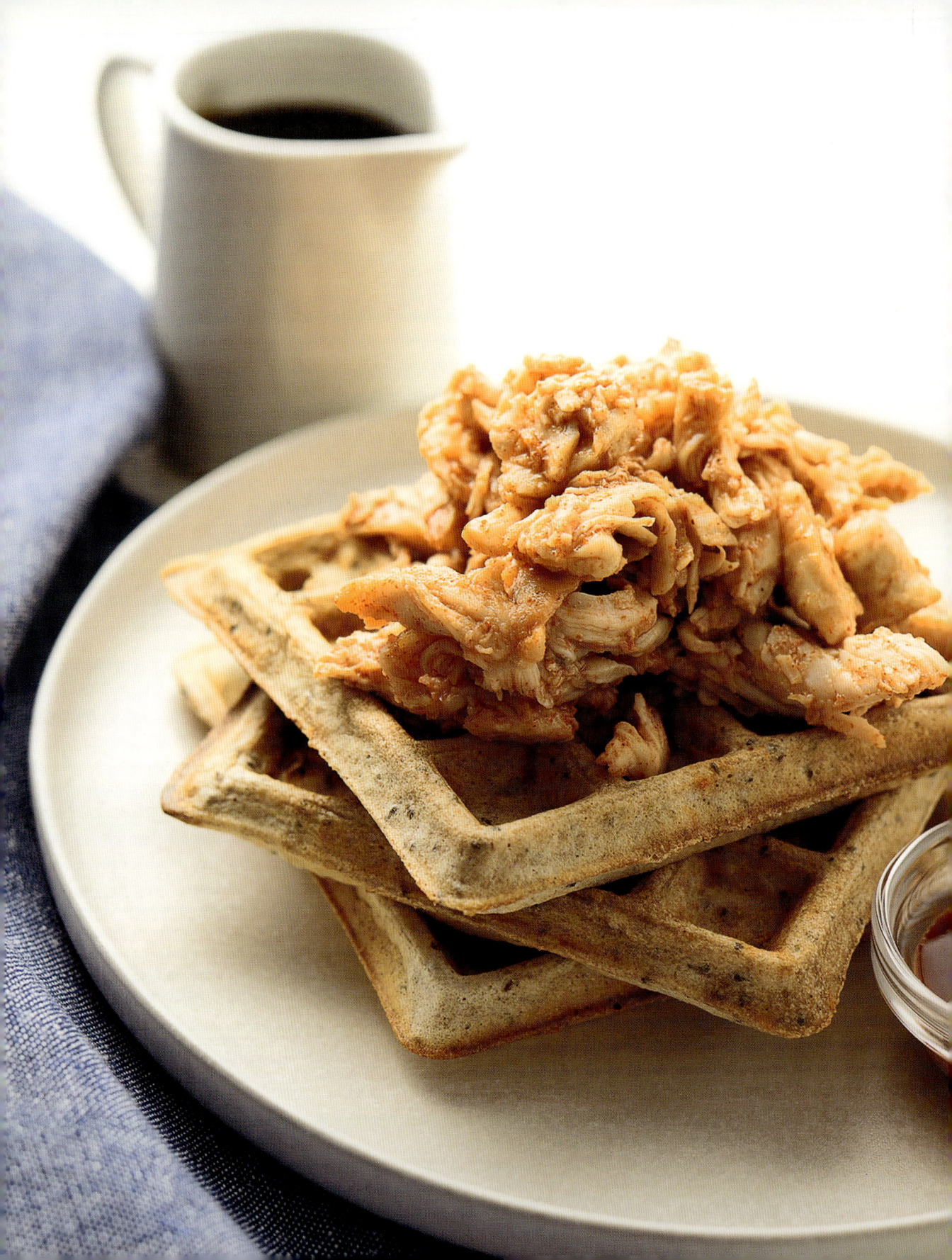

CHICKEN AND WAFFLES

■ **YIELD:**
1 SERVING

■ **PREP TIME:**
5 MINUTES

■ **COOK TIME:**
10 MINUTES

One important aspect of successfully lowering your cholesterol levels (and keeping them there) is figuring out how to continue enjoying your favorite foods in a more heart-healthy way. For my family, chicken and waffles is high on our favorites list, but low on the ideal-for-cholesterol list. That is—until we make it at home! Using high-fiber waffle mix and skipping the fried chicken, this meal definitely satisfies the craving for chicken and waffles without sacrificing our pursuit of lower levels. This recipe makes just a single serving, but can easily be increased to feed a crowd or prep a few meals in advance.

FOR THE WAFFLE

½ cup (53 g) high-protein pancake mix, such as Kodiak Buttermilk Power Cakes

⅓ cup (80 ml) soy milk or low-fat milk

¼ cup (60 ml) egg whites

¼ teaspoon ground cinnamon

1 tablespoon (11 g) chia seeds

1 teaspoon olive oil

Nonstick cooking spray

FOR THE CHICKEN

⅔ cup (150 g) shredded cooked chicken

1 tablespoon (15 ml) hot sauce

2 teaspoons maple syrup

TO MAKE THE WAFFLE

Plug in a waffle iron or heat a medium skillet over medium heat. In a medium bowl, mix the pancake mix, soy milk or low-fat milk, egg whites, cinnamon, chia seeds, and olive oil together until combined. The dough should be thicker than pancake batter.

Spray the waffle maker or skillet with nonstick cooking spray. Pour mixture into a waffle iron or make a large pancake in a skillet. Cook for 3 minutes on each side, or until golden brown.

TO MAKE THE CHICKEN

While the waffle is cooking, add chicken, hot sauce, and maple syrup to a small skillet over medium heat until bubbly and warmed through. Stir occasionally. Alternatively, you can combine the ingredients in a microwavable bowl and microwave on high until warm, about 1 minute.

When the waffle is finished cooking, remove it from the waffle iron or skillet and add it to a serving plate. Top with spicy chicken and enjoy!

NUTRITIONAL ANALYSIS

SERVING SIZE: 1 waffle + ⅔ cup (about 150 g) chicken

PER SERVING: 457 calories; 18 g fat; 2 g saturated fat; 41 g protein; 33 g carbohydrate; 6 g dietary fiber

SWEET POTATO AND SAUSAGE HASH

Made in the microwave, this meal is easy to make, fast to cook, and big on flavor. Does microwaving your food impact its nutritional quality? No! This is a common misconception. Microwaving is actually one of the best ways to preserve water-soluble nutrients in foods because they break down with prolonged exposure to heat. Microwaves work by creating friction inside the food that creates heat (just like if you were to rub your arm and it heats up). This heat then spreads throughout the food via a process called conduction. No nutrients are destroyed in the microwave that would be saved on the stove or in the oven, so feel free to whip up this simple sweet potato hash and enjoy it guilt-free.

■ **YIELD:**
1 SERVING

■ **PREP TIME:**
5 MINUTES

■ **COOK TIME:**
7 MINUTES

½ **large sweet potato, cubed**

½ **bell pepper, diced**

⅛ **red or white onion, diced**

1 **chicken or 1 tofurky sausage, sliced**

½ **cup (128 g) black beans**

¼ **teaspoon oregano**

¼ **teaspoon garlic powder**

⅛ **teaspoon salt**

⅛ **teaspoon ground black pepper**

Add sweet potato to a microwave-safe dish and microwave on high for 3 minutes. Add bell pepper and onion to the dish and microwave for 2 more minutes. Finally, add sausage, beans, and seasonings and stir. Microwave for another 2 minutes.

When finished cooking, use care to remove dish from microwave. It will be hot! Serve and enjoy.

NOTES

- Microwaving potatoes is an excellent way to cook them when you are crunched for time. Try the Loaded Baked Potato (page 93) in the dinner chapter too!

- Processed meats are a category of foods that should be enjoyed sparingly. While they may not be high in saturated fat, very high intakes of processed meats are associated with an increased risk of high blood pressure, heart disease, and diabetes. Having them occasionally does not increase the risk, so enjoy them sparingly, not weekly.

NUTRITIONAL ANALYSIS

SERVING SIZE: ½ sweet potato + 1 sausage + ½ cup (128 g) black beans

PER SERVING: 393 calories; 10 g fat; 2 g saturated fat; 25 g protein; 53 g carbohydrate; 14 g dietary fiber

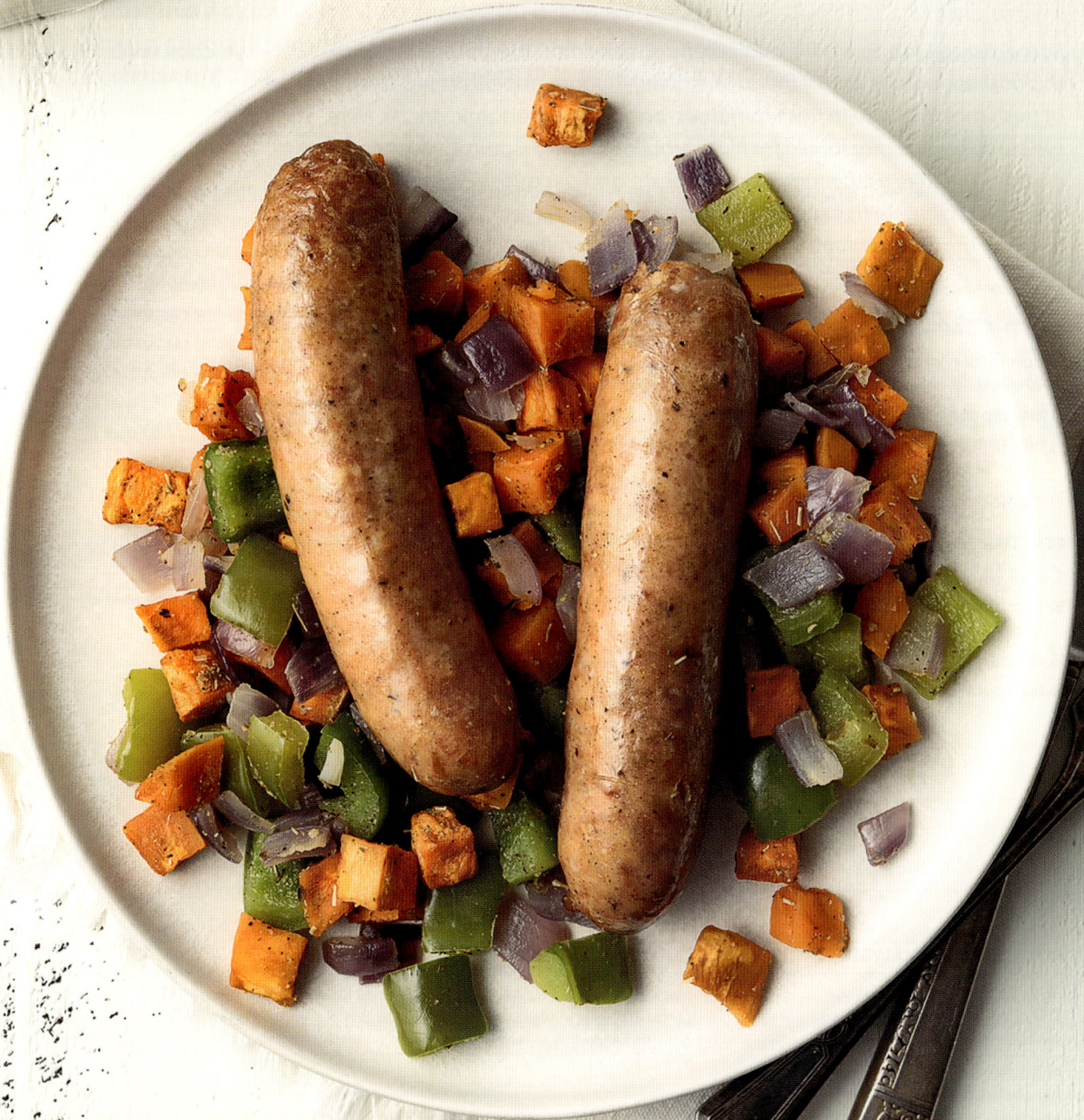

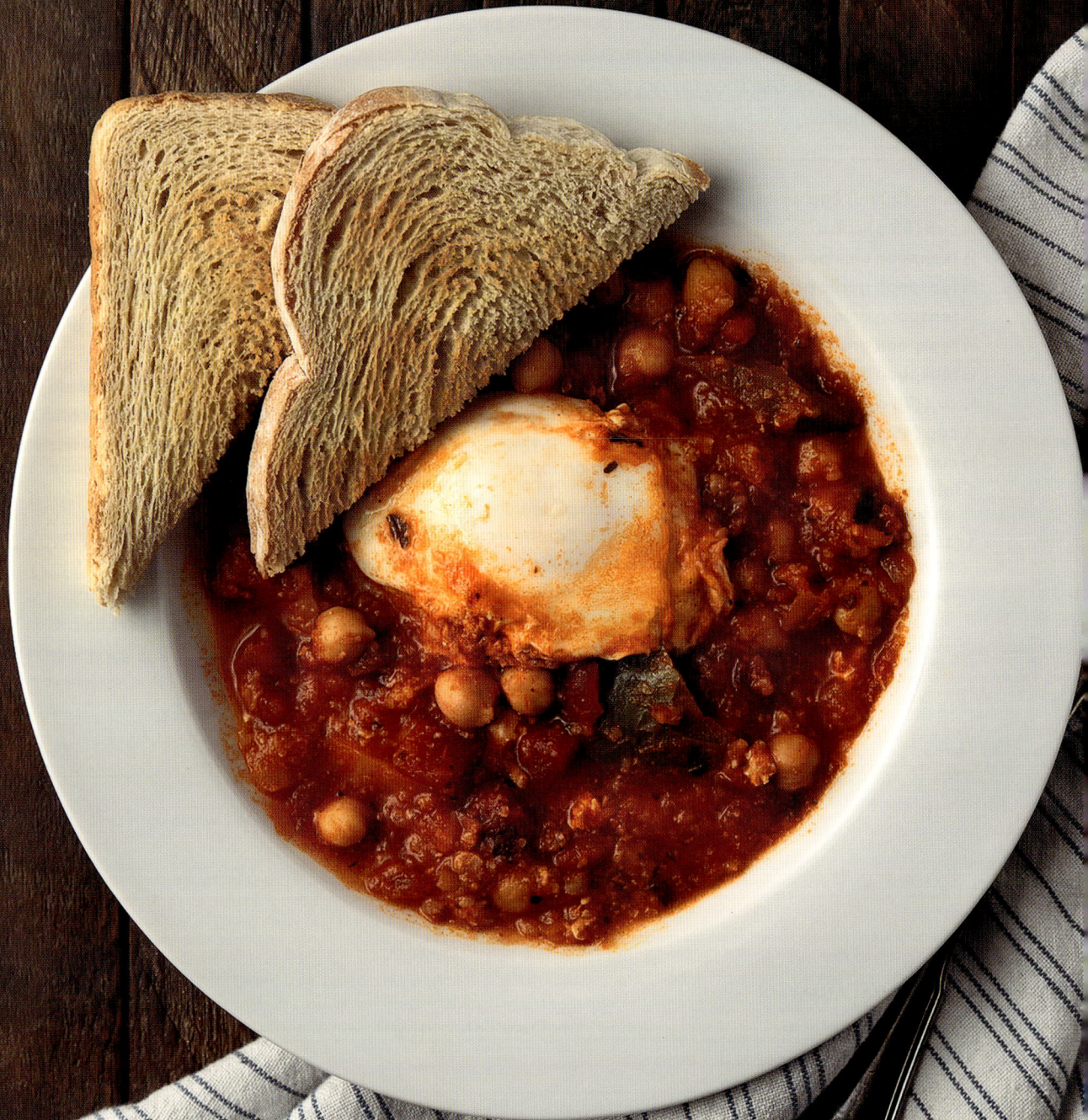

CHICKPEA SHAKSHUKA

A staple of Middle Eastern cuisines, shakshuka is an aromatic tomato-based dish with soft-cooked eggs and served with pita or crusty bread. My version has extra vegetables and chickpeas for added fiber without sacrificing on the flavor. Topped with feta cheese, it feels decadent while still supporting your cholesterol levels.

■ YIELD:
4 SERVINGS

■ PREP TIME:
0 MINUTES

■ COOK TIME:
15 MINUTES

1 tablespoon (15 ml) olive oil

½ cup (80 g) frozen onions

1 cup (150 g) frozen bell peppers

1 cup (132 g) frozen cauliflower (florets or riced)

1 (15.5-ounce [423 g]) can chickpeas, drained and rinsed

2 cups (490 g) no-sugar-added marinara sauce

4 eggs

¼ cup (30 g) feta cheese, divided

4 slices whole-grain bread, toasted

Heat olive oil in a medium sauté pan over medium-high heat. Add onions, bell peppers, and cauliflower, and sauté until tender, about 5 minutes. Add in chickpeas and marinara sauce. Stir to combine and turn heat down to medium-low. Make 4 wells in the mixture and crack an egg into each. Cover and allow to simmer until desired egg consistency is reached, about 6 to 8 minutes.

Divide the shakshuka between 4 plates. Each plate should have 1 egg and about one-quarter of the chickpea mixture. Serve garnished with 1 tablespoon (7 g) feta per serving and a piece of toast.

NUTRITIONAL ANALYSIS

SERVING SIZE: 1 egg + ¼ sauce + 1 slice toast

PER SERVING: 358 calories; 16 g fat; 4 g saturated fat; 20 g protein; 40 g carbohydrate; 10 g dietary fiber

NOTE

You can omit the feta cheese to reduce the saturated fat of this recipe down to 2 grams per serving.

OATMEAL (SWEET)

One of the biggest complaints I hear from people about oatmeal is that it doesn't keep them full for long and they get hungry for their next meal in just an hour or two. That's because they don't make their oatmeal satisfying enough by including plenty of healthy fats and a significant amount of protein. Trust me, oatmeal done right is very filling!

■ **YIELD:**
1 SERVING

■ **PREP TIME:**
0 MINUTES

■ **COOK TIME:**
10 MINUTES

½ cup (40 g) rolled oats

1½ cups (355 ml) soy or 0–2 percent milk

½ teaspoon vanilla extract

¼ teaspoon ground cinnamon

1 tablespoon (7 g) hemp hearts

1 tablespoon (11 g) chia seeds

1 tablespoon (16 g) nut or seed butter of choice, such as peanut, almond, or sunflower seed

This is my base oatmeal recipe that I make several mornings each week. I've included a list of suggested toppings and combinations you can try at the end of the recipe. Or improvise with your own preferred toppings, nut butters, or spices.

Add oats and milk to a small saucepan and place over medium-high heat. Add any extras you're including at this time for your desired variation (see Suggested Combinations) and stir to combine. Bring oatmeal to a gentle boil, then reduce the heat to medium-low and simmer, uncovered, for 5 minutes or until the oats have absorbed all of the liquid, stirring occasionally.

Remove oatmeal from the heat and add vanilla, cinnamon, hemp hearts, chia seeds, and nut butter. Top with desired fixings (see Suggested Combinations) and serve immediately.

SUGGESTED COMBINATIONS

- Peanut Butter and Jelly: Use peanut butter and top with homemade berry chia jam (see Peanut Butter and High-Fiber Jam Sandwich, page 86).

- Banana Bread: Top with ½ sliced banana and 2 tablespoons (15 g) chopped walnuts.

- Pumpkin Pie: Add ¼ cup (61 g) canned pumpkin when cooking oats and substitute pumpkin spice blend for the cinnamon.

- Carrot Cake: Add ¼ cup (28 g) shredded carrots when cooking oats. Add ⅛ teaspoon each nutmeg, cloves, and dried ginger. Top with 2 tablespoons (18 g) raisins and 1 tablespoon (8 g) chopped walnuts.

- Dessert: Add 1 tablespoon (5 g) cocoa powder and 1 teaspoon maple syrup. Top with 1 tablespoon (11 g) dark chocolate chips.

NUTRITIONAL ANALYSIS (base recipe)

SERVING SIZE: About 1 cup (about 200 g) oatmeal

PER SERVING: 490 calories; 25 g fat; 3 g saturated fat; 25 g protein; 41 g carbohydrate; 11 g dietary fiber

OATMEAL (SAVORY)

Most people have only ever eaten oatmeal as a sweet breakfast. For people who don't like sweets in the morning, oatmeal can be a nonstarter. This savory oatmeal recipe is a great alternative and still packs the nutritional punch of sweeter oatmeal. Use the base recipe below and add your favorite savory toppings. I've included some suggestions to get you started.

■ **YIELD:**
1 SERVING

■ **PREP TIME:**
0 MINUTES

■ **COOK TIME:**
10 MINUTES

½ cup (78 g) rolled oats

1 tablespoon (10 g) chia seeds

1½ cups (425 ml) chicken or beef bone broth

1 whole egg or ¼ cup (60 ml) egg whites

¼ teaspoon garlic powder

¼ teaspoon onion powder

⅛ teaspoon ground black pepper

SUGGESTED TOPPINGS

Green onions

No-sugar-added sunflower seed butter

Sautéed mushrooms

Shredded chicken

Soft-boiled egg

Add oats, chia seeds, and bone broth to a small saucepan over high heat. Bring oatmeal to a gentle boil, then reduce the heat to medium-low and simmer for 5 minutes or until the oats have absorbed all of the liquid, stirring occasionally. Turn off the heat. Crack the egg into a ramekin or measure out egg whites. Slowly pour egg or egg whites into the oatmeal while rapidly stirring the oats to prevent scrambling of the egg. Keep mixing for 2 minutes before adding the garlic powder, onion powder, and black pepper.

Serve your savory oatmeal in a bowl with the topping of your choice.

NUTRITIONAL ANALYSIS (base recipe)

SERVING SIZE: About 1 cup (about 200 g) oatmeal

PER SERVING: 320 calories; 12 g fat; 3 g saturated fat; 26 g protein; 32 g carbohydrate; 8 g dietary fiber

NOTES

- The egg gives this oatmeal a very creamy consistency, like a pudding.

- Bone broth is similar to broth or stock, but typically made over a longer period of time and with some acid to break down the bones used in cooking. This provides more protein per serving just from the cooking liquid. If you cannot find bone broth, regular broth works just fine.

- The saltiness of the oatmeal will depend on the salt content of the bone broth. If using a no-salt-added bone broth, add ⅛ teaspoon salt to the broth before cooking or add a drizzle of soy sauce before serving.

- Use a more nutritious cooking liquid than water to make sweet or savory oatmeal. Milk or bone broth adds about 8 grams of additional protein per cup (235 ml) (and they taste better too)!

BERRY SMOOTHIE

A smoothie is an excellent option to get a lot of nutrition into a portable and time-efficient meal. You may have heard a rumor that fiber disappears when blended. This is false. Fiber does not go anywhere when blended into a smoothie. It may break down into smaller fragments, but its impact on the body is exactly the same. And while we're debunking myths, here's another: Blended fruit does not spike your blood sugar levels more than eating a whole fruit. Enjoy your smoothie guilt-free!

YIELD:
1 SMOOTHIE

PREP TIME:
5 MINUTES

COOK TIME:
0 MINUTES

1 cup (150 g) frozen berries, such as blueberries, raspberries, or mixed berry blend

2 tablespoons (32 g) nut butter of choice, such as peanut, almond, or sunflower seed

½ cup (115 g) 0 percent Greek yogurt

1 cup (235 ml) water

⅛ teaspoon ground cinnamon

Vanilla protein powder, enough to add 10 g of protein

Add all of the ingredients except the protein powder to a blender. Blend on high for about 45 seconds to thoroughly combine. Remove the lid and add protein powder. Blend on low for 15 seconds until combined. Pour into your favorite glass or to-go cup and enjoy.

NOTES

- Feel free to add vegetables to this smoothie, such as frozen spinach or frozen cauliflower. You have lots of opportunities to add vegetables throughout your day, though, so don't feel pressured to add them to your smoothies unless you want to!

- Are protein powders okay for lowering cholesterol? Yes, absolutely. Just be mindful of the amount of saturated fat per serving. Unflavored protein powders should have 0 grams. If it is a whey or casein powder, it will have some dietary cholesterol, but that is okay. Ideally, added sugars will be less than 5 grams per serving. I recommend just one serving of protein powder or protein bars per day since they don't often provide the other benefits of nutrients from food.

NUTRITIONAL ANALYSIS

SERVING SIZE: 1 smoothie

PER SERVING: 375 calories; 16 g fat; 3 g saturated fat; 30 g protein; 30 g carbohydrate; 7 g dietary fiber

PUMPKIN SMOOTHIE

In my opinion, pumpkin should be enjoyed all year long. It is one of the best sources of beta-carotene, one of the key antioxidants that can help to reduce inflammation in the body. This shake is creamy, thick, and delicious. Feel free to enjoy it in any season!

■ **YIELD:**
1 SMOOTHIE

■ **PREP TIME:**
5 MINUTES

■ **COOK TIME:**
0 MINUTES

½ cup (123 g) pureed pumpkin (about ⅓ can)

1 date, pitted

½ teaspoon pumpkin spice

2 handfuls ice

1 tablespoon (10 g) chia seeds

1¼ cups (295 ml) soy milk or 0–2 percent milk

Vanilla protein powder, enough to add 10 g of protein

Add all ingredients except protein powder to the blender. Blend on high for 60 to 90 seconds, or until you no longer hear the ice being crushed. Once blended, remove the top and add protein powder. Blend on low for 15 seconds until combined. Serve immediately.

NOTES

- You'll want to drink this smoothie right away. The chia seeds will begin to thicken the smoothie as soon as it is finished blending!

- Why add the protein powder separately? Most protein powders contain whey, which is often used in food processing because it has a range of food science applications. One of them is as a foaming agent. When blended for 90 seconds, whey protein will cause large bubbles to form in smoothies, especially at the top. Gently blending it in will ensure that it doesn't change the consistency of the smoothie.

NUTRITIONAL ANALYSIS

SERVING SIZE: 1 smoothie

PER SERVING: 407 calories; 12 g fat; 1 g saturated fat; 34 g protein; 38 g carbohydrate; 8 g dietary fiber

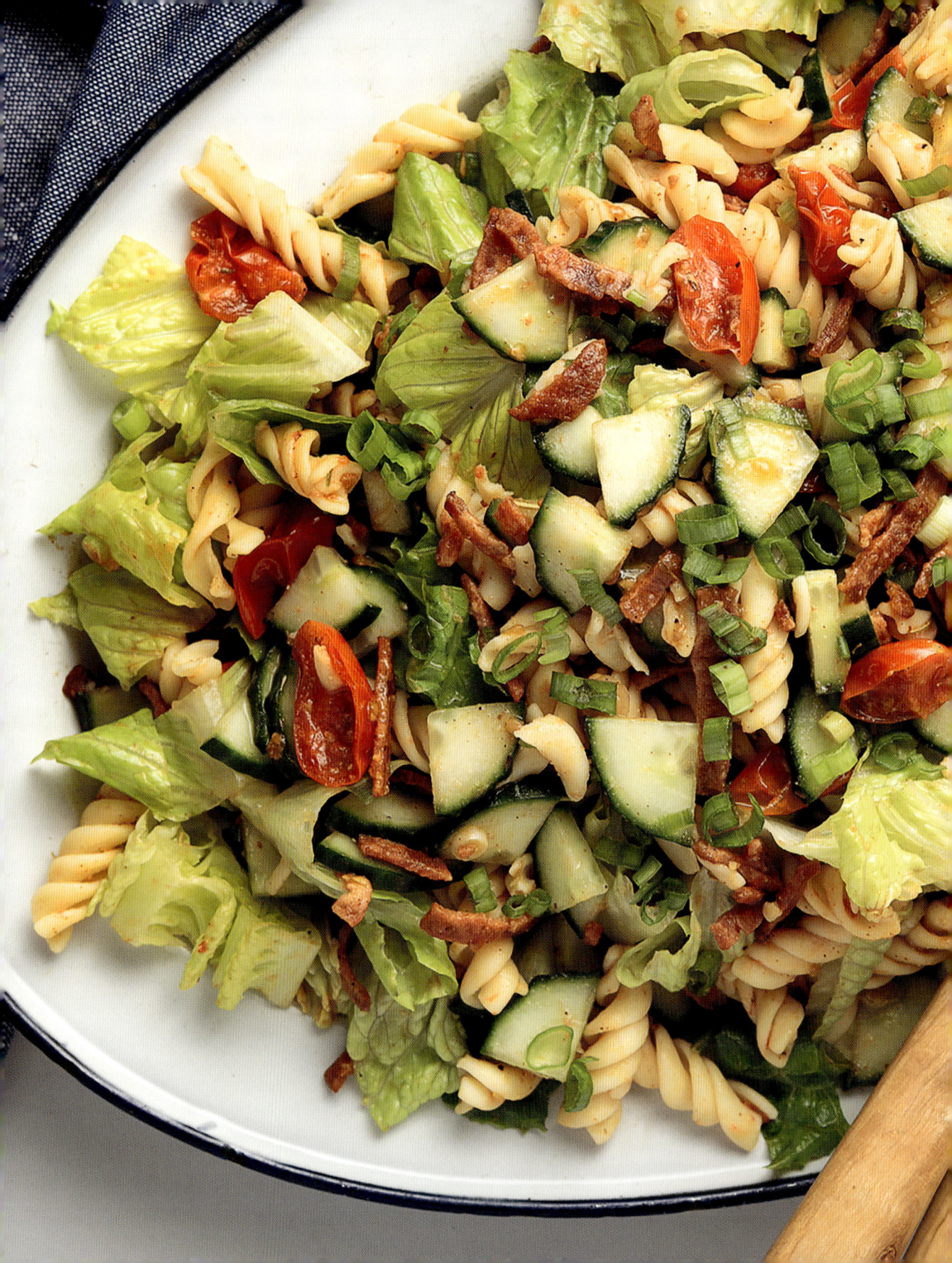

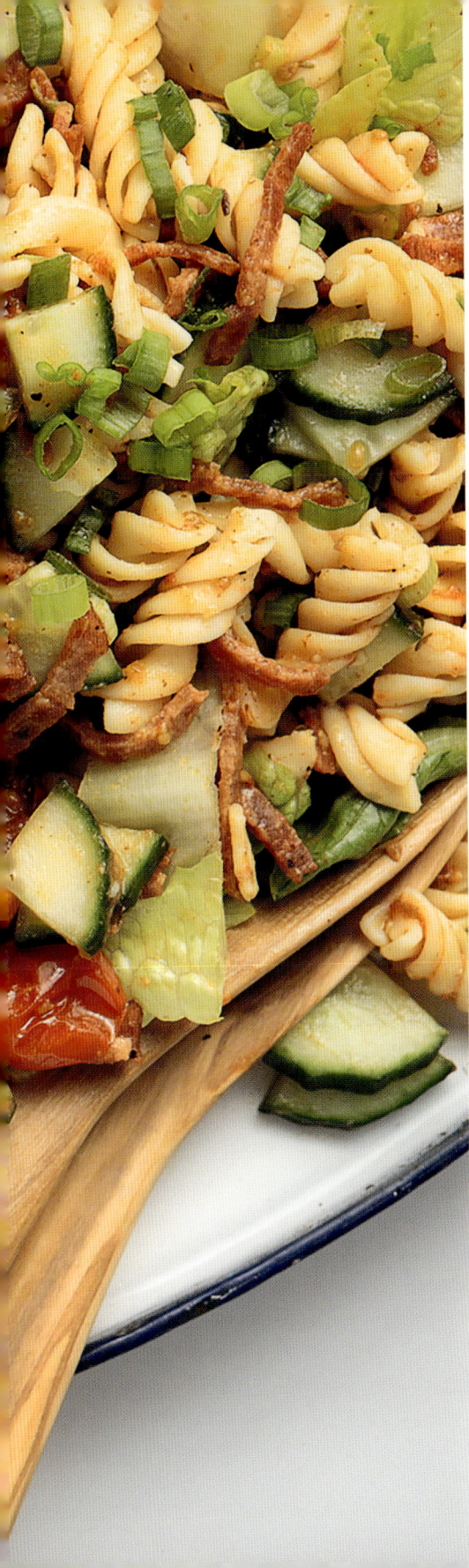

CHAPTER 4

20 Lunches in 20 Minutes

Based on my experience with my clients, lunch often just happens without much planning. Whether it is grabbing something quick while running between meetings, digging in the snack drawer at the office or home, or throwing together random things from the refrigerator, there seems to be a lack of forethought on ensuring that lunch is nutritious and balanced. My strategy involves a combination of dinner leftovers, easy throw-together options, and two dedicated lunch recipes each week to make lunch something you look forward to that also helps you hit your nutrient goals. Equally important is carving out enough time to eat it without distraction during the day!

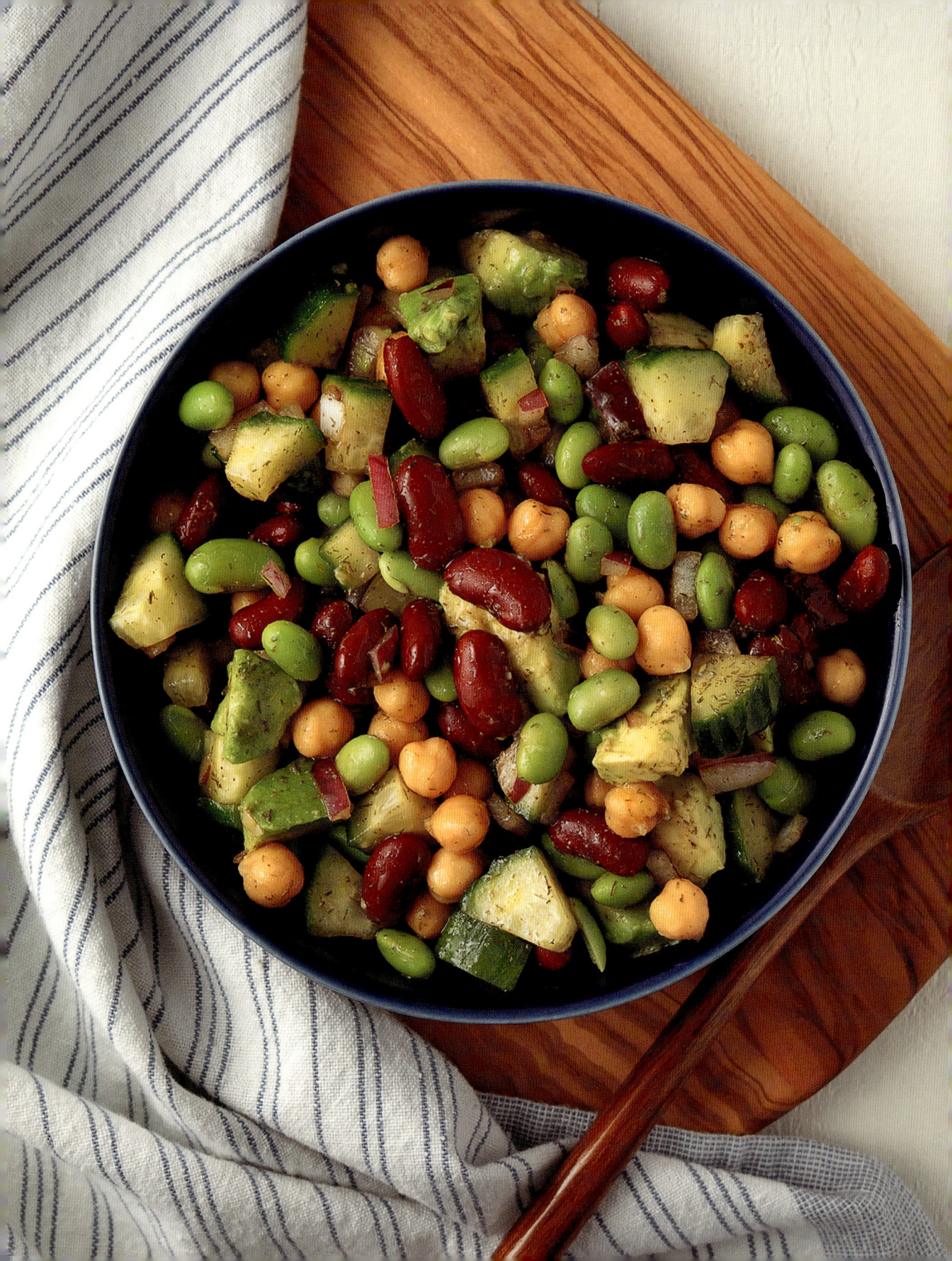

THREE-BEAN SALAD WITH EDAMAME

This hearty bean salad only gets better the longer the ingredients sit, making it an awesome lunch to prep for the week. The combination of textures and flavors makes this dish unique, plus the fiber and protein in the beans will keep you full for hours and help you meet your daily fiber goal.

■ YIELD:
4 SERVINGS

■ PREP TIME:
10 MINUTES

■ COOK TIME:
0 MINUTES

1 avocado, cubed

1 teaspoon lime or lemon juice

2 cups (340 g) shelled edamame

1 (15.5-ounce [423 g]) can kidney beans, drained and rinsed

1 (15.5-ounce [423 g]) can chickpeas, drained and rinsed

1 English cucumber, cubed

¼ red onion, finely diced

2 tablespoons (28 ml) avocado oil

2 tablespoons (28 ml) rice vinegar

1½ tablespoons (25 ml) soy sauce

1 teaspoon ground cumin

½ teaspoon garlic powder

1 tablespoon (3 g) dried dill

Salt to taste

Fresh cilantro for garnish, optional

In a small bowl, toss cubed avocado in lemon or lime juice. Set aside.

Add remaining ingredients to a large bowl and mix to combine. Add avocado and gently toss to combine. Serve in a bowl, topped with cilantro, if using.

NOTES

- If making in advance, add avocado (about ¼ avocado per serving) the day you plan to eat.

- Looking for more protein? Canned tuna, salmon, or sardines are a tasty addition to this dish. Adding 2 ounces of fish provides about 15 grams of protein.

NUTRITIONAL ANALYSIS

SERVING SIZE: About 2½ cups (about 300 g) salad

PER SERVING: 455 calories; 18 g fat; 3 g saturated fat; 23 g protein; 52 g carbohydrate; 18 g dietary fiber

EASY CHOPPED SALAD JARS

■ YIELD:
1 SERVING

■ PREP TIME:
5 MINUTES

■ COOK TIME:
0 MINUTES

Assembling your daily salad in a jar not only saves you the mental effort of putting together lunch every day, but it keeps the salad ingredients fresh for you to enjoy up to a week after making them. Use the following recipe as a template, but make sure to follow the same order of ingredients to keep your ingredients fresh for days: dressing, beans, additional protein (plant or animal), onions, nuts or seeds, sturdy vegetables (like onion, carrot, and celery), then more delicate vegetables (like cucumbers and tomatoes), and finally, your salad greens.

1½ teaspoons olive oil

1 teaspoon Dijon mustard

½ teaspoon Italian seasoning

¼ teaspoon salt

⅛ teaspoon ground black pepper

¾ cup (180 g) chickpeas, drained and rinsed

2 tablespoons (20 g) red onion

2 tablespoons (20 g) pumpkin seeds

½ cup (70 g) chopped cucumber

½ cup (75 g) cherry tomatoes, halved

½ head romaine lettuce, diced

In a large quart-size mason jar, add ingredients in the order they are listed. The order prevents the last items from getting soggy. Try to keep the jar upright to prevent the dressing from spreading too early.

Remove from the refrigerator about 30 minutes before you are ready to eat to let the olive oil come back to room temperature (it will harden in the fridge). When you are ready to eat, vigorously shake the jar to evenly coat all of the ingredients in the dressing. Dump the salad onto a plate or into a bowl and enjoy.

NOTE

Want to add more protein? Add roughly 15 grams of protein by including 2 ounces (55 g) of cooked chicken or one-half a 5-ounce (140 g) can of tuna. These should be added after the chickpeas.

NUTRITIONAL ANALYSIS

SERVING SIZE: 1 salad jar

PER SERVING: 501 calories; 22 g fat; 3 g saturated fat; 26 g protein; 59 g carbohydrate; 23 g dietary fiber

EASY RAMEN WITH TOFU AND BROCCOLI

YIELD:
1 SERVING

PREP TIME:
0 MINUTES

COOK TIME:
10 MINUTES

This tofu ramen is another recipe that can be made with long-lasting ingredients that you may already have in your refrigerator and pantry. Made with frozen veggies, tofu, and dried ramen noodles, this dish is also the ultimate lunch meal that comes together in about 10 minutes. I typically make this dish with chicken broth, which gives it a "meaty" taste even though it's made with tofu.

- 1 (2-ounce [55 g]) cake brown rice ramen noodles
- ⅓ (15-ounce [420 g]) block firm tofu, cubed into bite-size pieces
- 1 cup (156 g) frozen broccoli or green beans
- 1½ cups (355 ml) chicken, vegetable, or beef broth
- 1 teaspoon soy sauce or coconut aminos
- ½ teaspoon fish sauce
- ½ teaspoon sesame oil

Add ramen noodles, tofu, frozen vegetables, and broth to a pan over medium-high heat. Bring to a boil. Begin to pull apart noodles with a fork. Reduce to a simmer and cook until noodles are tender, approximately 3 to 4 minutes, until noodles are soft and vegetables and tofu are warm.

Remove from heat and serve in a bowl topped with soy sauce or coconut aminos, fish sauce, and sesame oil.

NUTRITIONAL ANALYSIS

SERVING SIZE: 1 bowl ramen

PER SERVING: 428 calories; 13 g fat; 3 g saturated fat; 24 g protein; 52 g carbohydrate; 8 g dietary fiber

NOTE

Frozen shrimp or edamame are other easy options for this ramen. Follow the same instructions, but substitute 1 cup (170 g) frozen shrimp or 1 cup (170 g) frozen edamame for the tofu.

LEMONY CHICKEN SOUP

■ YIELD:
4 SERVINGS

■ PREP TIME:
5 MINUTES

■ COOK TIME:
15 MINUTES

You'll find yourself coming back to this refreshing soup recipe over and over again. This twist on chicken soup uses beans in place of noodles to add fiber and protein, while the lemon brightens the dish and makes even the coldest days seem a bit sunnier. Loaded with vegetables, it is a surprisingly filling soup that comes together in less than 20 minutes!

1 tablespoon (15 ml) olive oil

1 onion, diced

3 carrots, thinly sliced

2 celery stalks, thinly sliced

½ teaspoon salt

1 teaspoon dried rosemary

4 cups (950 g) chicken broth

1 bunch kale, chopped, about 4 cups (268 g)

2 (15.5-ounce [423 g]) cans white beans, drained and rinsed

2 cups (280 g) cooked shredded chicken breast, about ½ pound (225 g)

¼ cup (60 ml) lemon juice

In a large, deep sauté pan, heat olive oil over medium-high heat. Sauté onion, carrots, and celery with salt and rosemary until tender, about 10 minutes. Add chicken broth, kale, white beans, and chicken. Bring to a simmer. Turn off heat and add lemon juice. Stir to combine and serve.

NUTRITIONAL ANALYSIS

SERVING SIZE: About 2 cups (about 475 ml) soup

PER SERVING: 473 calories; 10 g fat; 1 g saturated fat; 40 g protein; 48 g carbohydrates; 17 g dietary fiber

NOTE

This dish tastes just as delicious without the chicken, but the protein content will decrease.

FREEZER STIR-FRY

This is perhaps the ultimate quick lunch option! Almost everything that you need for this meal can be kept in the freezer. I love making this dish when I don't have anything to take for lunch. I simply mix the ingredients together and take it with me to work. Store in the fridge and microwave it at lunchtime. It is a very low-effort lunch that still ticks all the nutrition boxes for lowering your cholesterol!

■ **YIELD:**
1 SERVING

■ **PREP TIME:**
5 MINUTES

■ **COOK TIME:**
5–10 MINUTES

1 teaspoon avocado oil,
  if making on stove

1 cup (156 g) frozen broccoli

½ cup (50 g) frozen brown rice

½ cup (85 g) frozen edamame

½ cup (65 g) frozen pea, corn,
  and carrot mix

1½ tablespoons (11 g) hemp
  seeds

1 tablespoon (16 g) sunflower
  seed or peanut butter

1 teaspoon soy sauce

¼ teaspoon garlic powder

TO MAKE IN THE MICROWAVE

Add everything to a glass storage container and give it a good shake to mix. Remove the lid and microwave for 2 minutes and 30 seconds. Re-cover and allow to sit for 2 minutes. Stir and enjoy!

TO MAKE ON THE STOVE

Add a splash of water or 1 teaspoon of avocado oil to a medium sauté pan. Add broccoli first, since it usually takes the longest to cook. Sauté for 2 to 3 minutes before adding brown rice, edamame, and mixed vegetables. Cook for 3 to 5 more minutes until they are thoroughly heated through. Turn off the heat and add hemp seeds, nut butter, soy sauce, and garlic powder. Stir to combine. Serve in a bowl and enjoy.

NOTES

- If your broccoli florets are very large, they might need more time in the microwave. I recommend cutting them into smaller pieces after about 1 minute in the microwave to speed up the cooking time.

- You can substitute any frozen vegetables that you have on hand in this recipe.

NUTRITIONAL ANALYSIS

SERVING SIZE: About 2½ cups
(about 350 g) stir-fry

PER SERVING: 478 calories; 20 g
fat; 2 g saturated fat; 23 g protein;
53 g carbohydrates; 12 g dietary fiber

TUNA OR SALMON NIÇOISE SALAD

The beauty of this not-so-fancy take on a tuna niçoise salad is that it can be made in advance. Using sturdy vegetables and canned fish, it will taste even better after a day marinating in the dressing.

■ **YIELD:**
2 SERVINGS

■ **PREP TIME:**
5 MINUTES

■ **COOK TIME:**
10 MINUTES

FOR THE SALAD

¼ pound (115 g) fingerling potatoes, halved

8 ounces (225 g) green beans or haricots verts, trimmed

2 eggs

1 (5-ounce [140 g]) can tuna or salmon packed in water, drained

½ cup (120 g) canned chickpeas, drained and rinsed

FOR THE DRESSING

2 tablespoons (22 g) whole-grain mustard (see Note)

2 tablespoons (28 ml) olive oil

1 teaspoon dried rosemary

1 garlic clove, finely chopped

⅛ teaspoon salt

⅛ teaspoon ground black pepper

TO MAKE THE SALAD

Add potatoes to a medium pot and cover with water. Bring to a boil over high heat and cook for 10 to 12 minutes, or until potatoes are tender. Add green beans during the final 2 minutes of cooking. Drain and rinse with cold water to stop the cooking process.

While the potatoes and green beans are cooking, add 2 eggs to a small saucepan. Cover with water and bring to a boil. Once boiling, turn off the heat and cover. Allow eggs to sit for 10 minutes. When the eggs are done, pour off hot water and shake eggs in the pan until they crack (this will make them easier to peel). Remove the eggs from the pan and submerge immediately in cold water to stop the cooking process. Peel and cut in halves.

TO MAKE THE DRESSING

While the potatoes and eggs are cooking, mix the dressing. Add all ingredients to a small jar and shake to combine. Set aside.

Assemble your salad on 2 plates and top with the dressing. This can be eaten immediately or stored for a few days in the refrigerator.

NUTRITIONAL ANALYSIS

SERVING SIZE: ½ assembled salad + 2 tablespoons (28 ml) dressing

PER SERVING: 519 calories; 22 g fat; 4 g saturated fat; 37 g protein; 43 g carbohydrates; 9 g dietary fiber

NOTE

You can substitute Dijon or spicy brown mustard if whole-grain mustard isn't to your taste.

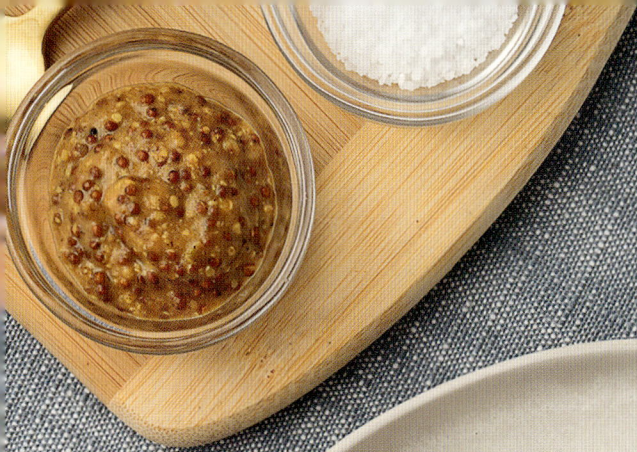

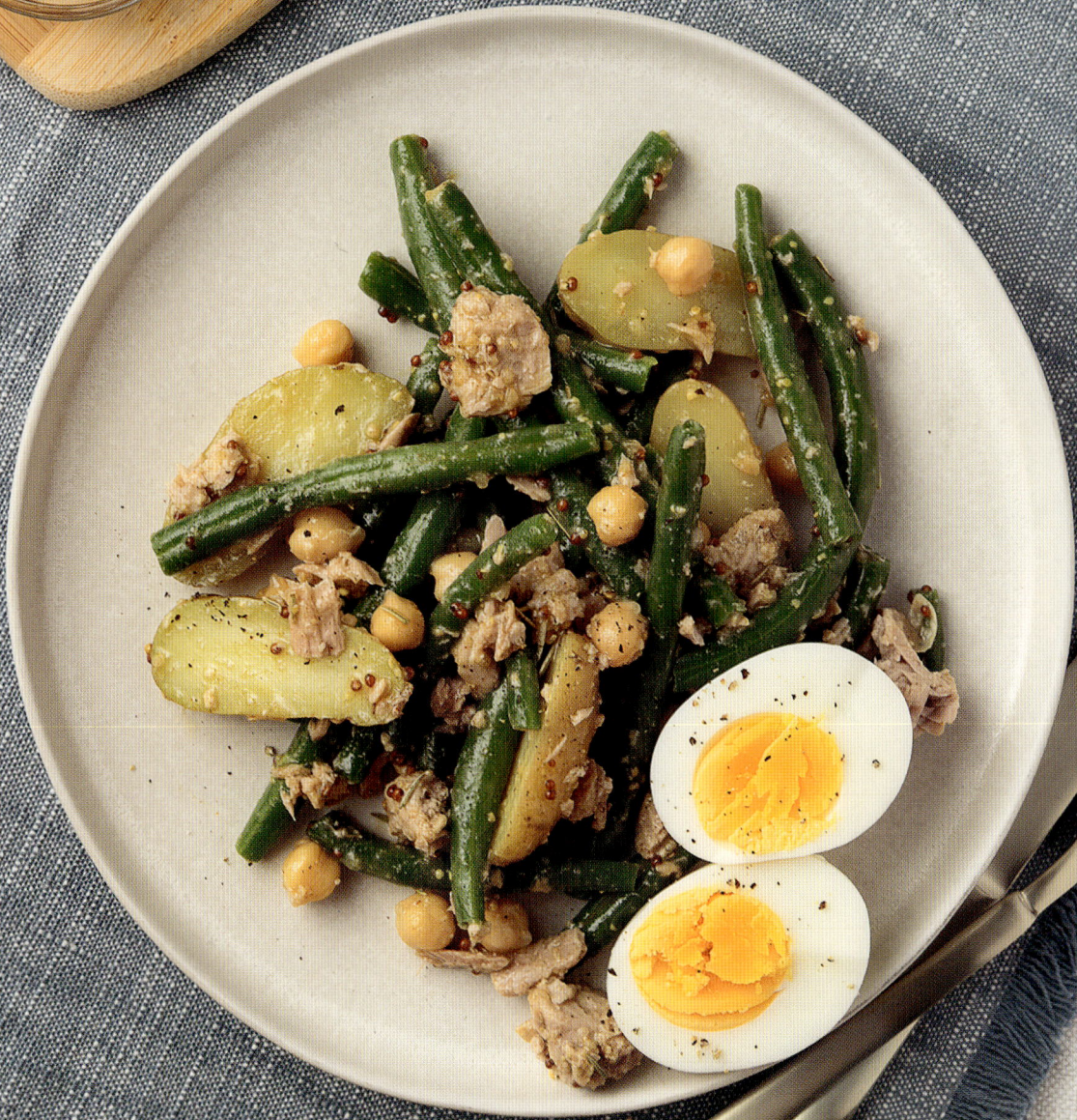

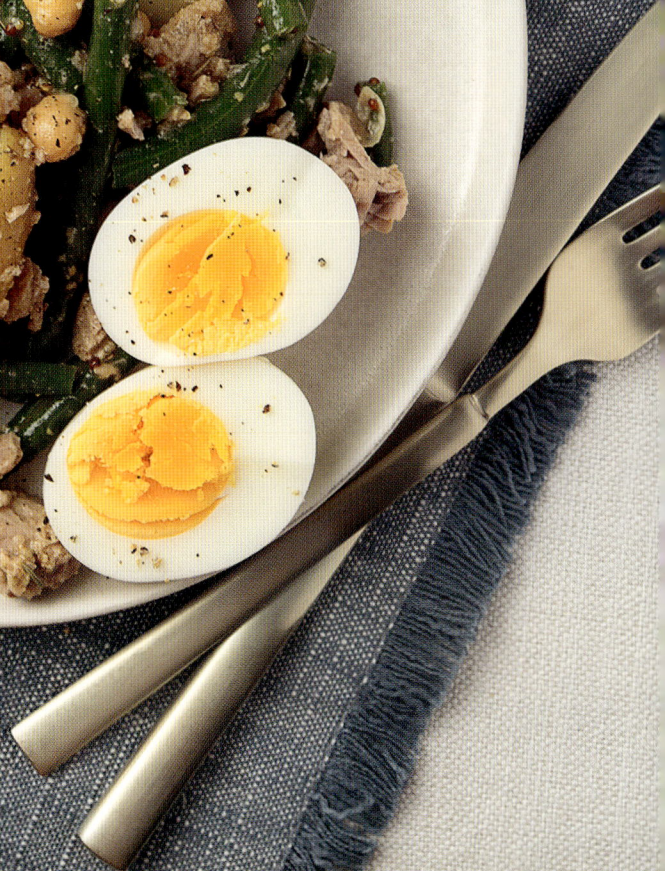

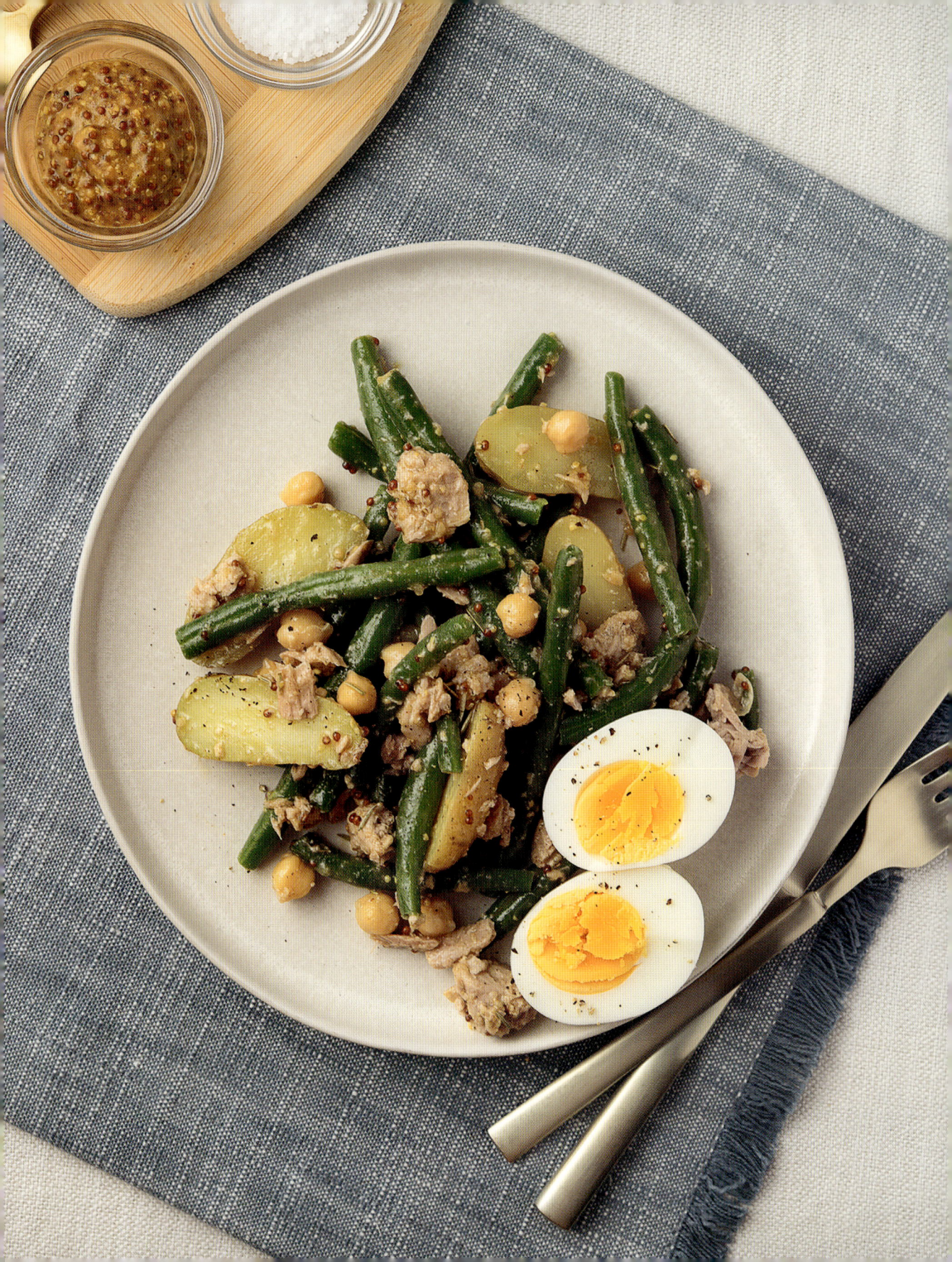

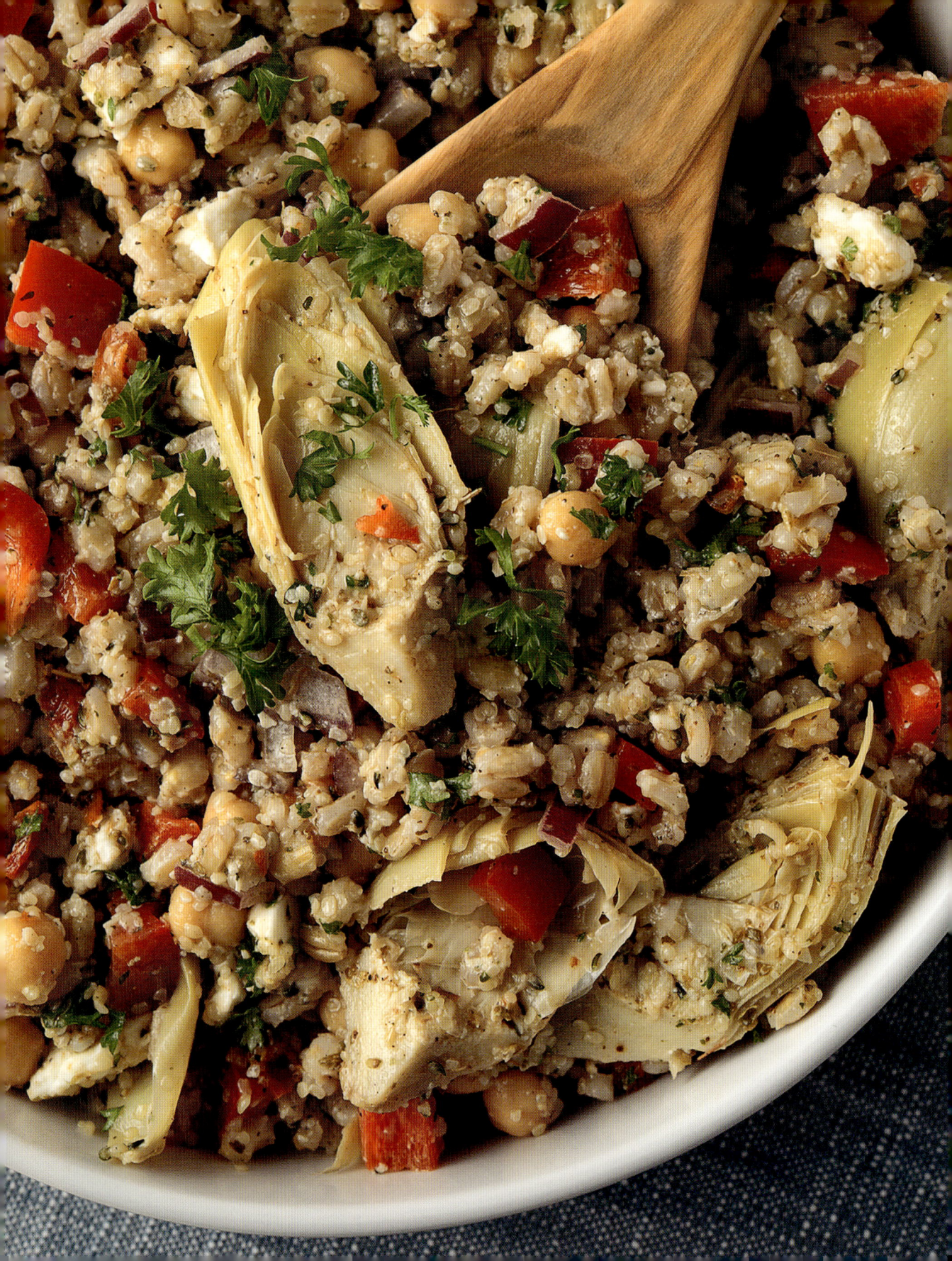

MEDITERRANEAN CHOPPED SALAD

■ YIELD:
4 SERVINGS

■ PREP TIME:
10 MINUTES

■ COOK TIME:
0 MINUTES

This is a hearty and dense salad that gets better the longer it sits. It's the perfect make-ahead lunch because all of the vegetables and grains can handle the dressing for a few days (unlike lettuce). Made with a soluble-fiber superstar, barley, that's high in beta-glucan, Mediterranean Chopped Salad is a winner for your tastebuds and your cholesterol.

1 (14-ounce [397 g]) can artichoke hearts, drained and chopped

1 (15.5-ounce [423 g]) can chickpeas, drained and rinsed

¼ cup (28 g) sun-dried tomatoes in oil, chopped

1 red bell pepper, diced

¼ red onion, finely diced

2 cups (314 g) cooked barley

¼ cup (15 g) fresh parsley, chopped

¼ cup (16 g) fresh oregano, chopped, or 1 tablespoon (3 g) dried oregano

2 tablespoons (28 ml) sun-dried tomato oil from the jar (see Notes)

¼ teaspoon salt

¼ teaspoon ground black pepper

Juice of ½ lemon

⅓ cup (50 g) crumbled feta cheese

¾ cup (90 g) hemp hearts

Toss artichoke hearts, chickpeas, sun-dried tomatoes, bell pepper, onion, and barley together in a large bowl until thoroughly mixed. In a separate small bowl, mix parsley, oregano, oil, salt, pepper, and lemon juice together. Pour the dressing over the barley mixture and toss to thoroughly combine. Gently toss in the feta cheese and hemp hearts. This salad can be enjoyed warm or chilled.

NUTRITIONAL ANALYSIS

SERVING SIZE: 2 cups (about 375 g) salad

PER SERVING: 470 calories; 23 g fat; 4 g saturated fat; 20 g protein; 50 g carbohydrates; 17 g dietary fiber

NOTES

- If your sun-dried tomato jar doesn't have enough oil, supplement with olive oil to reach 2 tablespoons (28 ml).

- Love a briny flavor? Remove the salt and add 2 tablespoons (17 g) capers, ¼ cup (25 g) sliced olives, or ¼ cup (60 g) sliced pepperoncini instead.

- Turkey pepperoni would be a good addition to this dish, but be mindful of the amount of processed meats you've consumed recently! Try to keep your intake of processed meats like bacon, sausage, deli meat, and charcuterie to 1 to 2 times per month. While these may not contribute much saturated fat, research shows that a high intake of processed meats is associated with an increased risk of high blood pressure, heart disease, and diabetes.

COLD NOODLE SALAD
WITH TOFU AND VEGGIES

■ **YIELD:**
3 SERVINGS

■ **PREP TIME:**
5 MINUTES

■ **COOK TIME:**
10 MINUTES

This is the perfect fast and filling meal, especially in warm weather. This cold noodle salad is my husband's most recommended meal, and I often have everything I need to throw it together even when we are running low on groceries. It's light, fresh, and won't leave you overly stuffed. Plus, it has fiber and the tofu provides heart-healthy isoflavones, a plant compound found primarily in soy products that may have antioxidant functions, and is associated with decreased incidence of heart disease.

3 (2-ounce [55 g]) cakes brown rice ramen noodles

1 tablespoon (15 ml) avocado oil

1½ teaspoons sesame oil

Juice of ½ lime (about 1 teaspoon [5 ml])

½ teaspoon sugar or honey

1½ tablespoons (25 ml) soy sauce

1½ teaspoons fish sauce

1 (15-ounce [420 g]) block extra-firm tofu, cut into ½-inch (1 cm) cubes

2 green onions, both green and white parts, diced

1 head romaine lettuce, diced

½ medium cucumber, cut into matchsticks

1 tablespoon (8 g) white or black sesame seeds, divided

Prepare the noodles according to package instructions or use the following instructions. Bring a pot of water to a boil. Place noodles in a large heatproof bowl and pour in the boiling water. Let them soak for 5 to 7 minutes or until the noodles are tender. Drain and rinse under cold water.

While water is boiling and noodles are soaking, prepare the rest of the salad. In the bottom of a large bowl, whisk together avocado oil, sesame oil, lime juice, sugar or honey, soy sauce, and fish sauce. Next, add in tofu, green onions, romaine, and cucumbers. Toss to evenly coat in the sauce.

When the noodles are finished, add to the tofu and vegetables. Toss to coat the noodles with the sauce and combine all the ingredients. Plate one-third of the mixture in a salad bowl and top with 1 teaspoon sesame seeds.

NOTES

- You can make this recipe with any fresh vegetables that you have in the refrigerator. It is a great recipe to use up any leftover veggies at the end of the week!

- If you don't have tofu or just don't like it, you can substitute 2½ cups (425 g) of edamame for the tofu. I like to keep frozen edamame stocked in the freezer. Simply soak the beans in hot water while making the dish.

NUTRITIONAL ANALYSIS

SERVING SIZE: ⅓ salad

PER SERVING: 351 calories; 16 g fat; 3 g saturated fat; 21 g protein; 34 g carbohydrates; 7 g dietary fiber

GREEK SALAD WITH QUINOA

■ YIELD:
4 SERVINGS

■ PREP TIME:
20 MINUTES

■ COOK TIME:
20 MINUTES

This salad features the delicious taste of a traditional Greek salad, but swaps the lettuce for high-protein and high-fiber quinoa. Without the lettuce, this is a perfect dish to make at the beginning of the week and enjoy for lunch all week long. Boost the protein even further by customizing with your favorite protein source.

FOR THE SALAD

1 cup (173 g) quinoa

1 medium cucumber, diced

1 green bell pepper, diced

2 large tomatoes, diced, or 1 cup (150 g) cherry tomatoes, halved

¼ red onion, finely diced

1 (15.5-ounce [423 g]) can chickpeas, drained and rinsed

FOR THE DRESSING

¼ cup (60 ml) olive oil

2 tablespoons (28 ml) red wine vinegar

2 tablespoons (28 ml) apple cider vinegar

1 tablespoon (3 g) Italian seasoning

1 teaspoon onion powder

1 teaspoon garlic powder

¼ teaspoon salt

¼ teaspoon ground black pepper

½ teaspoon red pepper flakes, optional

TO MAKE THE SALAD

Cook quinoa according to package instructions. Allow to cool while you prep the vegetables.

In a large bowl, combine cucumber, bell pepper, tomatoes, red onion, and chickpeas. Add cooled quinoa and toss to combine.

TO MAKE THE DRESSING

In a small bowl, combine dressing ingredients and whisk together. Pour over salad, toss to coat, and serve.

NOTES

- This tastes even better the next day because the veggies and quinoa soak up the dressing.

- Looking for more protein? Add 2 ounces (55 g) cooked chicken or shrimp for about 15 grams of additional protein.

NUTRITIONAL ANALYSIS

SERVING SIZE: About 1½ cups (about 275 g) salad

PER SERVING: 423 calories; 18 g fat; 2 g saturated fat; 13 g protein; 54 g carbohydrates; 10 g dietary fiber

COBB PASTA SALAD

This pasta salad makes a perfect summertime dinner or make-ahead lunch. Filled with your favorite Cobb salad flavors, but much higher in fiber and lower in saturated fat than the traditional preparation, this recipe will become a staple in your lower-cholesterol journey.

■ **YIELD:**
3 SERVINGS

■ **PREP TIME:**
5 MINUTES

■ **COOK TIME:**
15 MINUTES

- 1 (8-ounce [225 g]) box bean-based pasta, like Banza
- 8 slices turkey bacon, thinly diced
- 2 tablespoons (28 ml) olive oil, divided
- 1 pint (340 g) cherry tomatoes, halved
- 2 tablespoons (22 g) spicy brown mustard
- 1 tablespoon (15 ml) red wine vinegar
- ¼ teaspoon salt
- ¼ teaspoon thyme
- ¼ teaspoon dried rosemary
- ¼ teaspoon garlic powder
- ¼ teaspoon ground black pepper
- 4 green onions, both green and white parts, thinly sliced
- ½ medium cucumber, sliced into half moons
- ⅔ head romaine lettuce, roughly chopped

Bring a large pot of water to a boil. Once boiling, add pasta and cook according to box instructions. Reserve ¼ cup (60 ml) cooking liquid. Drain the pasta and rinse with cold water when cooked. Set aside.

Cook turkey bacon in a skillet over medium-high heat with 1 tablespoon (15 ml) olive oil until crispy, about 5 minutes. Remove from skillet and set aside. Add cherry tomatoes to the pan with the remaining 1 tablespoon (15 ml) olive oil, mustard, vinegar, and seasonings. Cook until tomatoes are blistered and wilted, about 5 minutes. Add in turkey bacon and 2 tablespoons (28 ml) reserved pasta water. Stir and remove from heat.

Add cooled pasta to a large salad bowl and top with tomato-bacon mixture. Be sure to scrape the pot well to get all the sauce out. Next, top with green onions, cucumbers, and romaine lettuce. Toss and serve immediately.

To make in advance, store the green onions, cucumbers, and romaine separately. Add just before eating to main crispness.

NUTRITIONAL ANALYSIS

SERVING SIZE: 1½ cups (about 400 g) pasta salad

PER SERVING: 446 calories; 18 g fat; 1 g saturated fat; 29 g protein; 52 g carbohydrate; 9 g dietary fiber

NOTES

- Some bean-based pastas will boil over when cooking. To avoid the mess, add salt and cook in a large pot with plenty of extra room.
- Be mindful of your processed meat intake and try to limit it to two times per month.

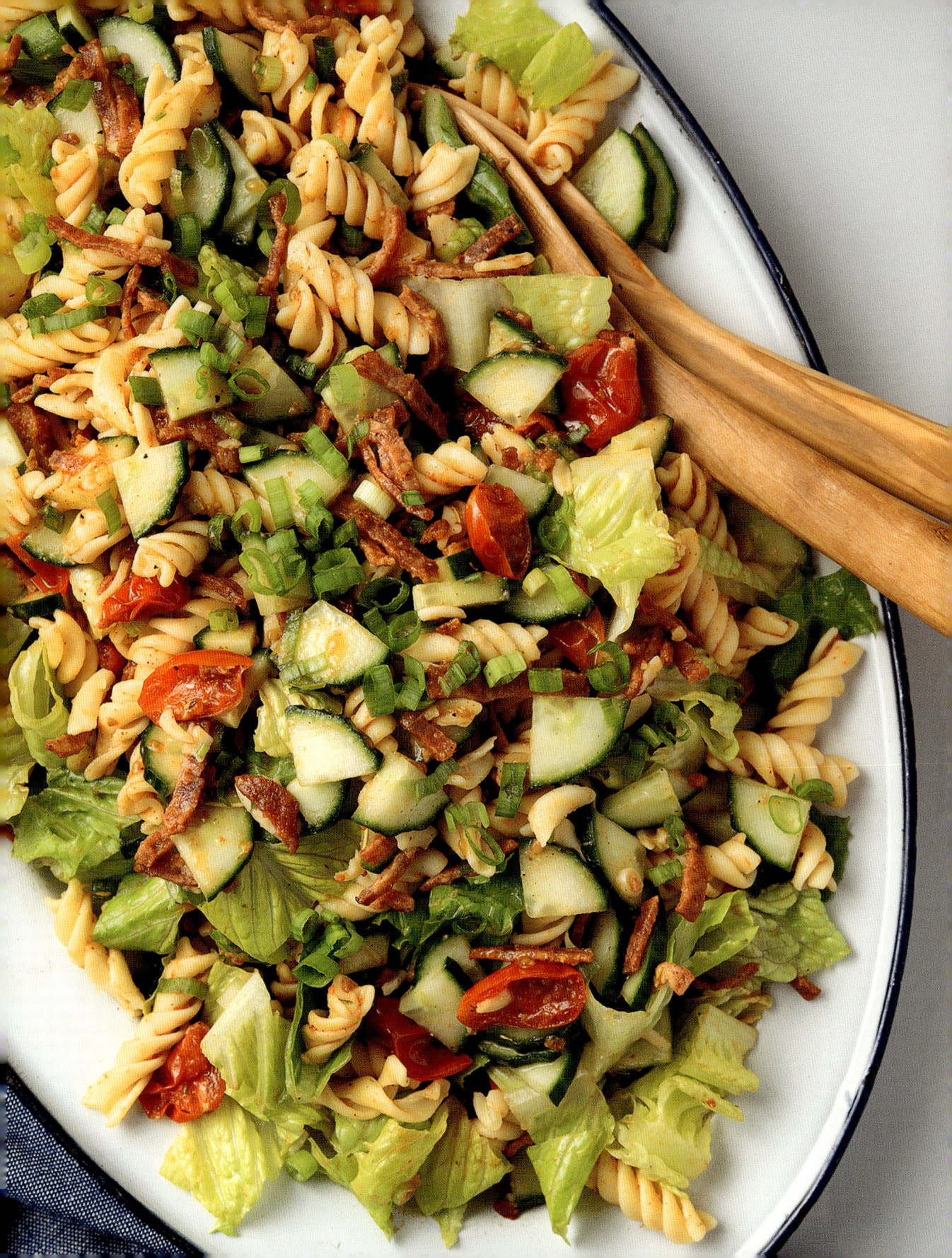

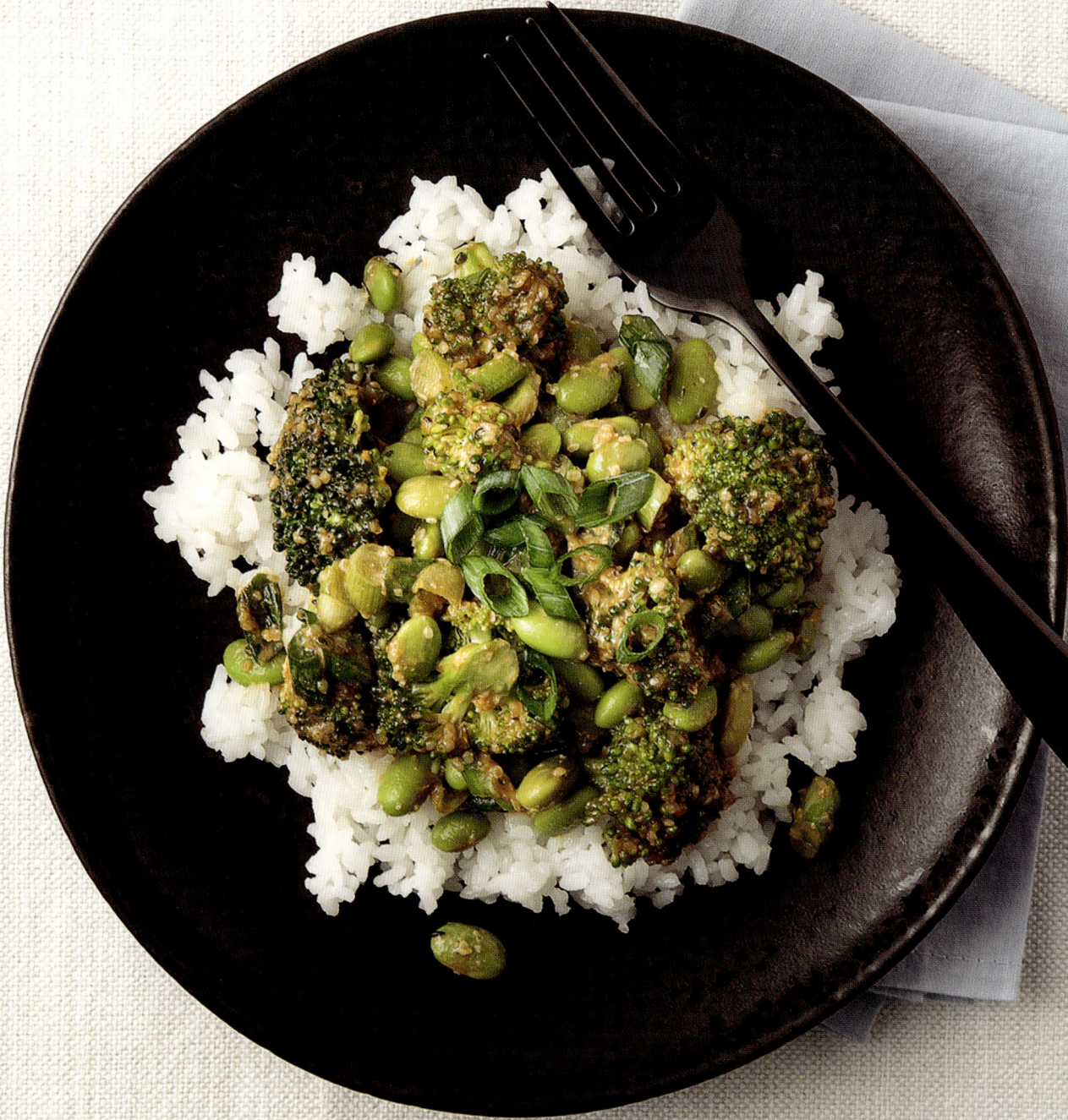

BROCCOLI HEMP SALAD

Packed with plant-based protein, antioxidants, and fiber, this Broccoli Hemp Salad is a powerhouse for both your tastebuds and your cholesterol. It's a salad you will return to often and is perfect as a side dish, over rice, or in a wrap.

■ **YIELD:**
4 SERVINGS

■ **PREP TIME:**
15 MINUTES

■ **COOK TIME:**
0 MINUTES

¼ cup (65 g) sunflower seed butter

1 tablespoon (15 ml) rice vinegar

2 tablespoons (28 ml) coconut aminos

1½ teaspoons soy sauce

1 tablespoon (15 ml) sesame oil

¼ cup (60 ml) water

1 garlic clove, minced

3 cups (468 g) broccoli florets, cut into bite-size pieces

3 cups (510 g) frozen edamame, thawed

4 green onions, both green and white parts, chopped

¼ cup (30 g) hemp seeds

Whisk sunflower seed butter, rice vinegar, coconut aminos, soy sauce, sesame oil, water, and garlic together in the bottom of a large bowl until a paste forms. Add broccoli, edamame, green onions, and hemp seeds. Give the salad a good toss to evenly coat all the ingredients in the dressing. Serve on its own in a bowl, in lettuce wraps, or over rice.

NUTRITIONAL ANALYSIS

SERVING SIZE: About 1½ cups (about 280 g) salad

PER SERVING: 373 calories; 21 g fat; 2 g saturated fat; 20 g protein; 26 g carbohydrates; 9 g dietary fiber

NOTES

- Not only is raw broccoli a good source of dietary fiber, but it is also a significant source of vitamin C with nearly 100 percent of your daily recommended intake per cup! Vitamin C is a key antioxidant to help manage inflammation.

- Sunflower seed butter is an excellent source of another antioxidant, vitamin E, with nearly 25 percent of your daily requirement in 1 tablespoon (16 g).

CHICKEN SALAD SANDWICH

Every kitchen needs a good chicken salad recipe, in my opinion. When made at home, chicken salad can absolutely fit into a nutrition plan for lower cholesterol levels. It is an excellent make-ahead lunch option that is always a crowd-pleaser.

■ **YIELD:**
1 SERVING

■ **PREP TIME:**
5 MINUTES

■ **COOK TIME:**
0 MINUTES

- 1 tablespoon (15 g) 0 percent Greek yogurt
- 1 tablespoon (14 g) mayonnaise
- 1 tablespoon (11 g) Dijon or whole-grain mustard
- 1 teaspoon seasoning blend of choice (see Notes)
- ⅔ cup (93 g) cooked shredded chicken breast
- 1 celery stalk, finely diced
- 1 green onion, both green and white parts, finely diced
- 2 slices 100 percent whole wheat bread or 15 seed-based crackers (see Notes)
- 6 carrot sticks or 1 cup (71 g) raw broccoli

In a medium bowl, stir together yogurt, mayonnaise, mustard, and seasoning. Add chicken, celery, and green onion. Toss until thoroughly coated. Spread the chicken salad on one slice of bread and top with the other to make a sandwich. Serve alongside raw vegetables.

NOTES

- Yes, you see mayonnaise in this recipe! While it is not a food that I recommend eating in large amounts all of the time, 1 tablespoon (14 g) mayonnaise has about 1.5 grams of saturated fat. Over the course of the day, that is maybe 10 percent of your saturated fat allowance. In this recipe, it's the same amount of saturated fat as the chicken. Chicken salad just tastes better with mayonnaise, in my opinion. Keep your intake in perspective for your entire day instead of thinking it needs to be eliminated 100 percent of the time.

- You can also substitute chickpeas for the chicken in this dish. Mash ¼ cup (60 g) of chickpeas and mix with the yogurt and mayonnaise. Then add another ¼ cup (60 g) of whole chickpeas with the celery and onion.

- Seasoning blends are usually a mixture of spices that taste good on basically everything. Some well-known ones are Old Bay, Season-All, or Kinder's All Purpose, to name a few.

- Mary's Gone Crackers is my recommended brand for seed-based crackers, but feel free to sub in your favorite.

NUTRITIONAL ANALYSIS

SERVING SIZE: 1 sandwich + vegetables

PER SERVING: 488 calories; 20 g fat; 3 g saturated fat; 37 g protein; 39 g carbohydrate; 9 g dietary fiber

SPANISH BLACK BEAN SOUP

■ **YIELD:**
4 SERVINGS

■ **PREP TIME:**
5 MINUTES

■ **COOK TIME:**
25 MINUTES

This soup was inspired by a black bean soup that I had at a Spanish restaurant a few years ago. It was smoky, hearty, and delicious. Most of the flavor in this soup comes from the chorizo. Chorizo is a heavily seasoned pork sausage. Pork sausage is not an ingredient that I would typically recommend for lowering cholesterol, but this recipe uses just 1 ounce per serving and provides so much delicious flavor that even the biggest meat eaters will love this bean-heavy dish. As a bonus, the soup has almost 20 grams of fiber per serving!

1 tablespoon (15 ml) avocado oil

1 medium red onion, diced

2 carrots, peeled and thinly sliced

2 celery stalks, thinly sliced

1 large red bell pepper, diced

1 teaspoon salt

1 teaspoon smoked paprika

4 ounces (115 g) ground Mexican chorizo

2 (15.5-ounce [423 g]) cans black beans, drained and rinsed, divided

2 cups (450 ml) chicken or vegetable stock

1 (15.5-ounce [423 g]) can diced tomatoes

1 tablespoon (1 g) fresh cilantro, optional

Coat the bottom of a deep sauté pan with avocado oil over medium heat. Add onion, carrots, celery, red bell pepper, salt, and smoked paprika. Sauté for 8 minutes or until vegetables begin to get tender. Add chorizo and cook for 5 minutes. Break meat into small bite-size pieces while cooking.

Add 1 can of black beans to a blender with chicken or vegetable stock. Blend on high for 15 seconds until beans begin to break down. Pour into the skillet with the remaining can of beans and the diced tomatoes. Bring to a simmer. To serve, ladle into a shallow bowl. Garnish with fresh cilantro, if using.

NUTRITIONAL ANALYSIS

SERVING SIZE: About 2 cups (about 450 g) soup

PER SERVING: 467 calories; 19 g fat; 5 g saturated fat; 23 g protein; 51 g carbohydrates; 19 g dietary fiber

NOTE

Mexican chorizo is fresh and ground, whereas Spanish chorizo is cured and smoked. Either will work in this dish. Mexican chorizo is often found behind the meat counter and Spanish chorizo is usually found in the precooked sausage section. If you can only find Spanish chorizo, remove the casing and finely dice to ensure the flavor gets into every bite. You should still add it at the same step, but the texture will be a bit tougher than Mexican sausage.

FISH TACOS

Fish tacos are a delicious and heart-healthy meal that combines fresh, flavorful ingredients with a cholesterol-friendly protein source. Topped with crunchy slaw, creamy avocado, and a zesty lime dressing, these tacos are packed with nutrients and are a great choice for your tastebuds and your heart.

■ **YIELD:**
1 SERVING

■ **PREP TIME:**
5 MINUTES

■ **COOK TIME:**
15 MINUTES

FOR THE FISH

1 teaspoon olive or avocado oil

1 teaspoon tomato paste

1 teaspoon chili powder

½ teaspoon garlic powder

½ teaspoon onion powder

Dash of salt

1 (5-ounce [140 g]) cod, halibut, or haddock fillet

2 corn tortillas

FOR THE AVOCADO SLAW

½ ripe avocado, cubed

¼ teaspoon salt

2 teaspoons lime juice

1 cup (90 g) shredded cabbage

1 tablespoon (10 g) red onion, finely diced

1 tablespoon (1 g) fresh cilantro

TO MAKE THE FISH

Preheat oven to 400°F (200°C or gas mark 6). Line a baking sheet with parchment paper.

Mix olive oil, tomato paste, chili powder, garlic powder, onion powder, and salt together into a paste. Rub the paste all over both sides of the fish. Bake for 10 minutes, then add corn tortillas in the oven directly on the top rack of the oven and bake for 2 to 3 more minutes until the fish is cooked through and flaky and reaches an internal temperature of 145°F (63°C).

TO MAKE THE AVOCADO SLAW

While the fish is baking, mix the ingredients for the avocado slaw in a medium bowl.

To serve, plate the corn tortillas. Separate the fish into flakes and evenly divide it between the 2 tortillas. Top with the slaw.

NOTE

Fish is the best source of omega-3s, which are essential nutrients that must come from the diet. Omega-3s play a crucial role for all of our cells, but particularly cells in the eyes and brain. They are also important for heart health. There are three different forms of omega-3s: eicosapentaenoic acid (EPA), docosahexaenoic acid (DHA), and alpha-linolenic acid (ALA). EPA and DHA can be found only in marine sources, like fish. ALA is found in some plants like walnuts, flaxseed, and chia seed. Fatty cold-water fish, like halibut, salmon, and mackerel, are great sources.

NUTRITIONAL ANALYSIS

SERVING SIZE: 2 tacos

PER SERVING: 428 calories; 19 g fat; 2 g saturated fat; 33 g protein; 37 g carbohydrates; 12 g dietary fiber

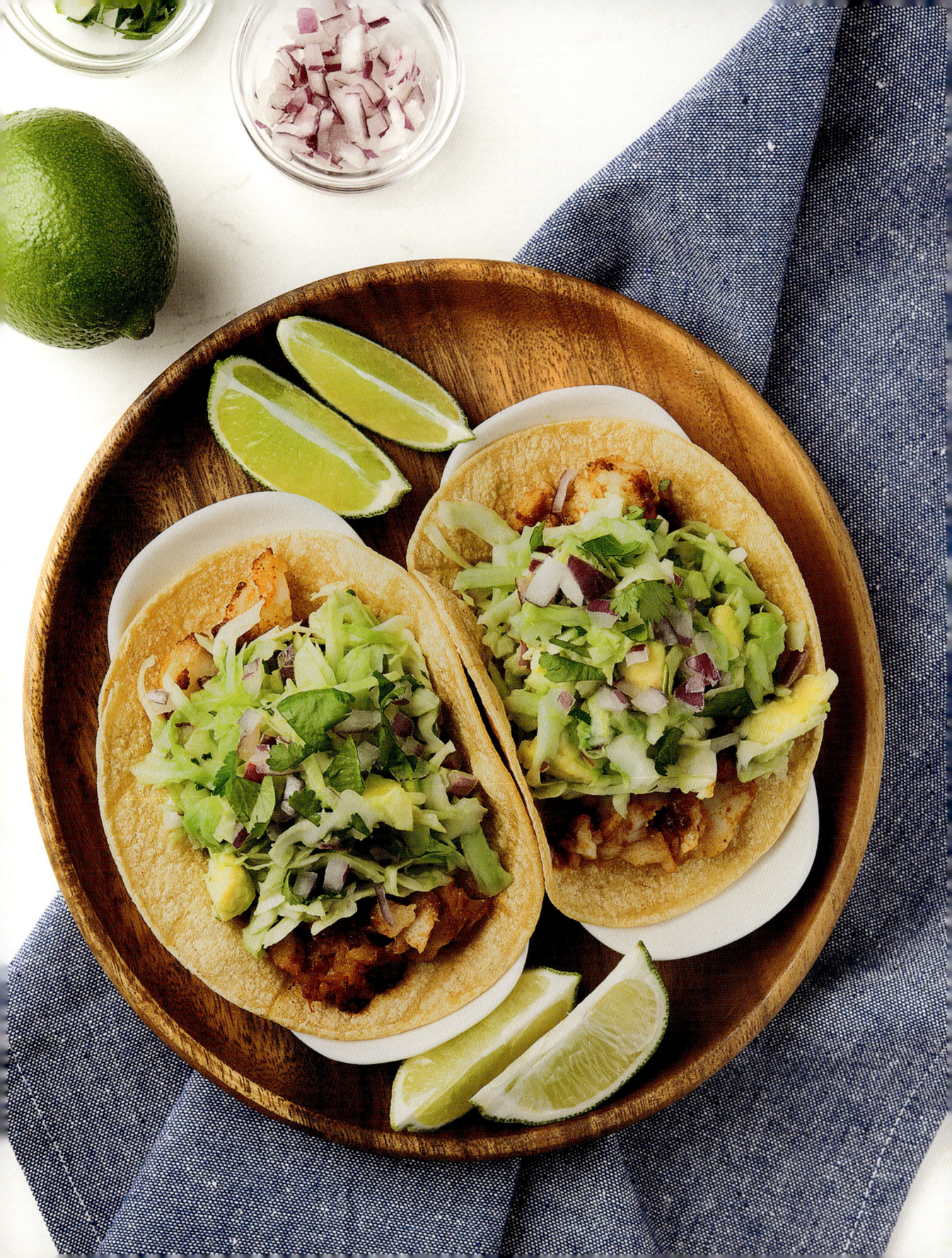

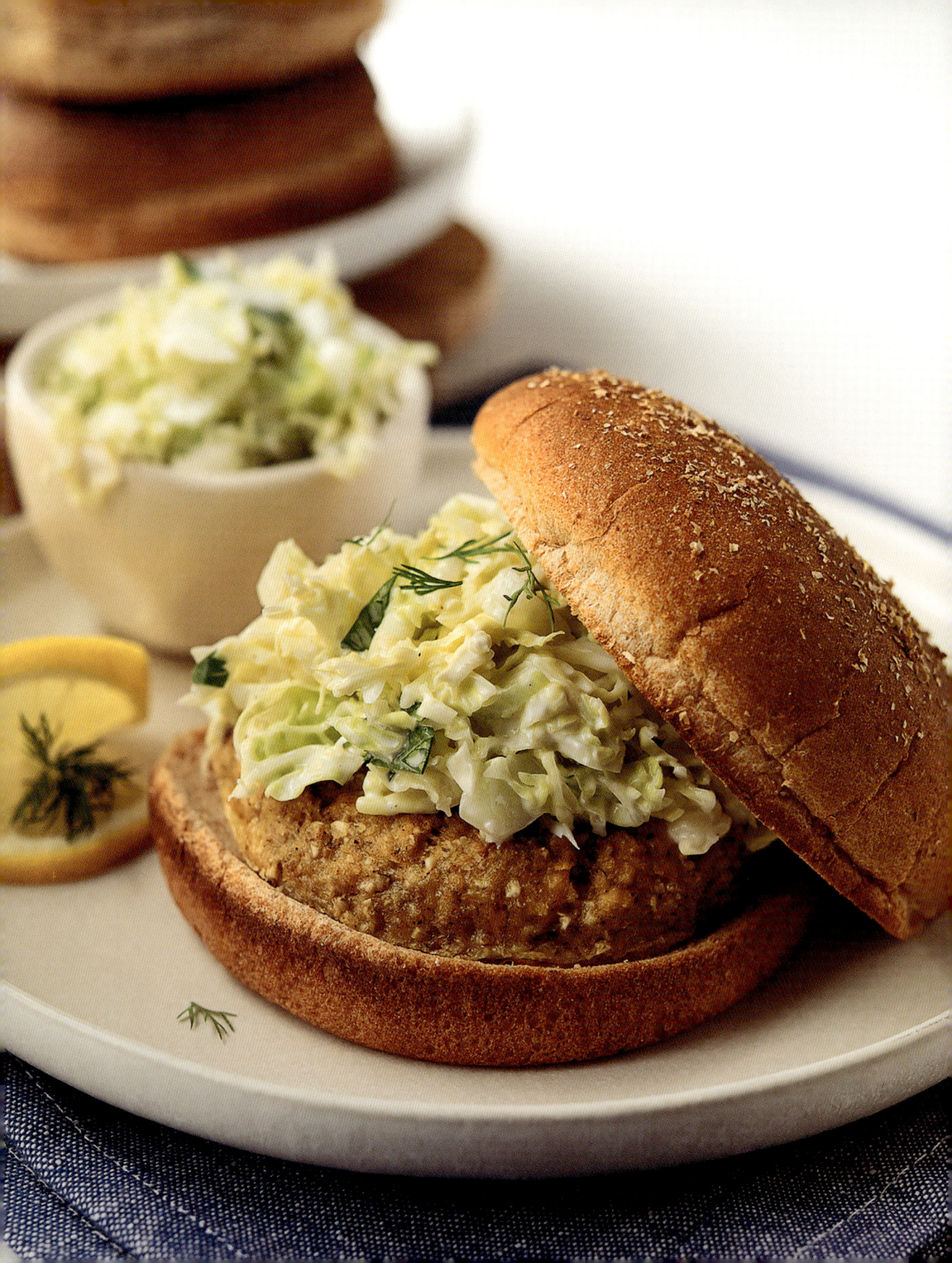

SALMON BURGER WITH CELERY SLAW

■ YIELD:
2 SERVINGS

■ PREP TIME:
5 MINUTES

■ COOK TIME:
10 MINUTES

Topped with a creamy slaw, these salmon burgers will quickly become a part of your weekly lunch rotation. Salmon is an excellent source of heart-healthy omega-3s, but preparing fresh salmon every week is not always realistic. This recipe uses shelf-stable canned salmon as a shortcut so you can get your omega-3s in no time.

FOR THE BURGERS

1 (6-ounce [140 g]) can pink salmon (see Notes)

1 egg, whisked

¼ cup (28 g) oat flour or bread crumbs

¼ teaspoon salt

¼ teaspoon ground black pepper

¼ teaspoon garlic powder

½ teaspoon onion powder

¼ teaspoon dill

2 whole wheat buns

FOR THE SLAW

1 celery stalk

1 cup (90 g) shredded cabbage

2 tablespoons (30 g) 0 percent Greek yogurt

1 tablespoon (14 g) mayonnaise

1 tablespoon (15 ml) lemon juice

⅛ teaspoon salt

⅛ teaspoon ground black pepper

Fresh cilantro, optional

NUTRITIONAL ANALYSIS

SERVING SIZE: 1 burger + ¼ cup (23 g) slaw

PER SERVING: 455 calories; 17 g fat; 4 g saturated fat; 37 g protein; 40 g carbohydrates; 6 g dietary fiber

TO MAKE THE BURGERS

Add canned salmon to a medium bowl and use a fork to break it up until there are no large chunks remaining. Add egg, oat flour or bread crumbs, salt, black pepper, garlic powder, onion powder, and dill. Use your hands to mix everything together. Form the mixture into 2 evenly sized burger patties. Add to the air fryer and cook for 6 minutes on 400°F (200°C) or until the internal temperature reaches 160°F (74°C). If you don't have an air fryer, coat a pan in nonstick spray and cook over medium-high heat for 4 minutes on each side.

TO MAKE THE SLAW

While the burgers are cooking, mix together slaw ingredients in a separate medium bowl and toast the whole wheat buns.

When burgers are finished cooking, assemble the burgers. Place the burger on the bottom bun, add half of the slaw, and top with the other half of the bun.

NOTES

- There are many types of canned salmon available. I find that wild pink salmon works the best for these salmon burgers. Sockeye salmon tends to be more expensive and has a stronger taste, although it does contain more omega-3s per serving.

- These burgers would taste delicious with many other spice combinations too. Try taco seasoning, curry blends, lemon pepper, or seafood seasoning. You likely won't need to add salt when using one of these blends, as it may contain salt already.

BBQ TEMPEH WRAPS

■ YIELD:
2 SERVINGS

■ PREP TIME:
10 MINUTES

■ COOK TIME:
10 MINUTES

Tempeh is made from soybeans that have been fermented. Tempeh has a firmer texture than tofu, but it still contains isoflavones, a plant compound found in soy that has been shown to lower the risk of coronary heart disease. Tempeh has a nutty flavor that pairs well with barbecue sauce, as well as Asian flavors—hence this BBQ wrap with marinated veggies!

1 (8.8-ounce [250 g]) package tempeh

⅓ cup (80 g) BBQ sauce of choice

1 teaspoon soy sauce

¼ teaspoon garlic powder

½ medium cucumber, sliced

½ cup (55 g) shredded carrots

⅛ red onion, thinly sliced

1 tablespoon (15 ml) rice wine vinegar

1 teaspoon sesame oil

2 whole wheat tortillas

2 leaves romaine lettuce, chopped

Fresh cilantro for garnish, optional

Slice tempeh into rectangular strips. Toss with BBQ sauce, soy sauce, and garlic powder in a large bowl. Add the strips to the air fryer on 400°F (200°C) and cook for 8 minutes or until crispy. If you don't have an air fryer, spray a medium pan with nonstick spray and cook the tempeh over medium heat for 4 to 5 minutes on each side or until it begins to get crispy.

While the tempeh is cooking, add cucumbers, carrots, and onion to a small bowl with vinegar and sesame oil and give them a gentle stir to coat. Let the veggies sit and marinate until the tempeh is done.

When the tempeh is cooked, assemble the wraps. Divide the tempeh evenly between the 2 wraps, placing them in a line in the center of each one. Top with lettuce, cucumber mixture, and cilantro, if using. To roll the wrap, fold one side over the tempeh. Next, tuck the ends and continue to roll until the wrap is sealed.

NUTRITIONAL ANALYSIS

SERVING SIZE: 1 wrap

PER SERVING: 496 calories; 13 g fat; 2 g saturated fat; 32 g protein; 66 g carbohydrates; 14 g dietary fiber

BUFFALO CHICKEN DIP

YIELD:
4 SERVINGS

PREP TIME:
5 MINUTES

COOK TIME:
0 MINUTES

This dip feels more decadent than it is. Swapping out the cream cheese for cottage cheese drastically reduces the amount of fat in the recipe without sacrificing creaminess or flavor. I love this dip as a sandwich, eaten with crackers, or as a dip for celery and carrot sticks. Because it comes together so quickly using cooked chicken, you have time to toss it in the oven and get the top bubbly and crispy too (see Notes).

---

1 cup (225 g) low-fat cottage cheese

¼ cup (60 ml) buffalo sauce

1 teaspoon garlic powder

½ teaspoon onion powder

¼ teaspoon ground black pepper

2 cups (280 g) cooked shredded chicken breast

3 celery stalks, thinly sliced

1 bunch green onions, both green and white parts, finely chopped

In a food processor or blender, combine cottage cheese, buffalo sauce, garlic powder, onion powder, and black pepper and blend until smooth. Combine sauce with chicken and vegetables in a medium bowl.

Serve your buffalo chicken dip on a sandwich, over a salad, or with high-fiber crackers or vegetables.

NUTRITIONAL ANALYSIS

SERVING SIZE: About ¾ cup (about 180 g) dip

PER SERVING: 198 calories; 6 g fat; 2 g saturated fat; 31 g protein; 6 g carbohydrates; 1 g dietary fiber

NOTES

- This dish also tastes delicious heated in the oven. Sauté the celery and onions before adding to the rest of the dip. Cook at 400°F (200°C or gas mark 6) for 15 minutes until bubbly.

- Without a vehicle to consume this dip, the fiber content is pretty low, so be sure to pair with a high-fiber bread, cracker, or veggie.

PEANUT BUTTER AND HIGH-FIBER JAM SANDWICH

■ YIELD:
1 SERVING

■ PREP TIME:
5 MINUTES

■ COOK TIME:
3 MINUTES

This is not your ordinary PB&J. With no added sugar and a fiber boost from the chia seeds, the high-fiber jam (made quick and easy in the microwave!) elevates this simple sandwich. You'll notice that there is saturated fat in this recipe. Like many other types of plants that contain fat, peanuts do contain some saturated fat. That does not mean that peanut butter needs to be eliminated (a question I receive often), but it is something to be mindful of when tallying your saturated fat total for the day.

¾ cup (109 g) frozen mixed berries

1 tablespoon (3 g) chia seeds

1 tablespoon (15 ml) water

2 slices 100 percent whole wheat bread

2 tablespoons (32 g) peanut butter

Place berries, chia seeds, and water in a microwave-safe bowl. Microwave for 2 minutes. Allow to cool in the microwave for 5 minutes while you prepare the rest of the sandwich.

Toast bread to your liking. Top one side of the bread with peanut butter. Once cooled, give the jam a stir and spread it onto the other piece of bread. Combine the 2 pieces into a sandwich. Enjoy!

NOTES

- Substitute sunflower seed butter or any other nut butter for the peanut butter.
- Serve with a side of vegetables, like sliced carrots, cucumbers, radishes, or tomatoes.

NUTRITIONAL ANALYSIS

SERVING SIZE: 1 sandwich

PER SERVING: 491 calories; 23 g fat; 4 g saturated fat; 19 g protein; 55 g carbohydrates; 12 g dietary fiber

OLIVE CHICKEN SANDWICH

If you think that chicken is boring, this chicken sandwich will change your mind! It is loaded with flavor, from the tangy chicken marinade to the olive tapenade. Your tastebuds will be very happy, and your heart will be too, because this meal is low in saturated fat, high in fiber, and packed with protein.

■ **YIELD:**
4 SERVINGS

■ **PREP TIME:**
5 MINUTES

■ **COOK TIME:**
15 MINUTES

FOR THE CHICKEN

1 pound (455 g) chicken breast, about 2 breasts

1 tablespoon (15 ml) olive oil

1 tablespoon (15 ml) red wine vinegar

¼ teaspoon ground black pepper

½ teaspoon salt

1 teaspoon oregano

FOR SERVING

4 whole wheat buns, toasted

¼ cup (65 g) jarred olive tapenade, divided

1 avocado, quartered

Red onion, thinly sliced

Lettuce leaves

1 cup (71 g) raw broccoli

6 carrot sticks

2 celery stalks, cut into sticks

TO MAKE THE CHICKEN

Slice each chicken breast lengthwise, halving the width of the chicken breast. Then, gently score each side of the breast meat by running your knife across the meat several times using light pressure so the knife doesn't go all the way through.

In a small bowl, mix together olive oil, vinegar, pepper, salt, and oregano. Add chicken and thoroughly coat with the marinade.

Heat a large skillet over medium-high heat. Add chicken to pan and cook for 7 minutes on each side or until it reaches an internal cooking temperature of 165°F (74°C).

TO SERVE

When the chicken is done, assemble your sandwiches. Spread 1 tablespoon (16 ml) olive tapenade on the bottom half of each bun. Next, mash ¼ of an avocado with a fork on top of the tapenade. Layer the sliced red onions and 1 to 2 lettuce leaves on top of the avocado, and top with one of the chicken breasts. Cover with the top of the bun and serve with broccoli, carrots, or celery.

NUTRITIONAL ANALYSIS

SERVING SIZE: 1 sandwich + 1 cup (about 70 g) raw veggies

PER SERVING: 416 calories; 16 g fat; 2 g saturated fat; 32 g protein; 34 g carbohydrates; 9 g dietary fiber

NOTE

Try batch cooking your protein for the week by doubling the chicken in this recipe. You can use it for any dish in this book that calls for "cooked chicken breast" like the Chicken and Waffles (page 49) or the Lemony Chicken Soup (page 66).

CHICKEN GYRO

A delicious spin on a take-out favorite, this chicken gyro will satisfy your craving without sacrificing your cholesterol. Made with ground flaxseed instead of eggs, and a whole wheat pita, this sandwich takes a bite out of your daily fiber needs. To mimic the texture of shawarma, the ground chicken is cooked in a log and then sliced. It is a delicious dish that comes together in about 20 minutes with the help of your trusty air fryer!

■ **YIELD:**
4 SERVINGS

■ **PREP TIME:**
5 MINUTES

■ **COOK TIME:**
15 MINUTES

FOR THE CHICKEN

1 pound (455 g) ground chicken or turkey

1 tablespoon (15 ml) olive oil

¼ cup (28 g) ground flaxseed

1 tablespoon (8 g) shawarma seasoning

1½ teaspoons salt

1½ teaspoons garlic powder

FOR THE SANDWICH

4 whole wheat pitas

¼ cup (60 g) store-bought tzatziki sauce, divided

1 head romaine lettuce, chopped

½ medium cucumber, thinly sliced

¼ red onion, finely diced

1 tomato, sliced

TO MAKE THE CHICKEN

Add ground chicken, olive oil, ground flaxseed, shawarma seasoning, salt, and garlic powder to a large bowl. Mix with your hands until thoroughly combined, then form into 4 evenly shaped cylinders or logs (think of a thick hotdog shape).

Cook the prepared chicken in an air fryer at 375°F (190°C) for 15 minutes or until an internal temperature of 165°F (74°C) is reached. If you do not have an air fryer, bake them in the oven at 375°F (190°C or gas mark 5) for 20 minutes. Once cooked, remove from the air fryer or oven and use a serrated knife to slice the logs lengthwise into 4 to 5 slices.

TO MAKE THE SANDWICH

To assemble the gyro, wrap the pitas in a damp paper towel and gently warm them in the microwave for 20 seconds. They can also be warmed in the air fryer or oven for just a few minutes. When the pitas are warm and pliant, spread 1 tablespoon (15 g) tzatziki evenly across the bottom half of each one. Then top with romaine, cucumber, red onion, and tomato. Top with sliced chicken. Fold in half and enjoy.

NUTRITIONAL ANALYSIS

SERVING SIZE: 1 gyro

PER SERVING: 451 calories; 19 g fat; 4 g saturated fat; 32 g protein; 43 g carbohydrates; 10 g dietary fiber

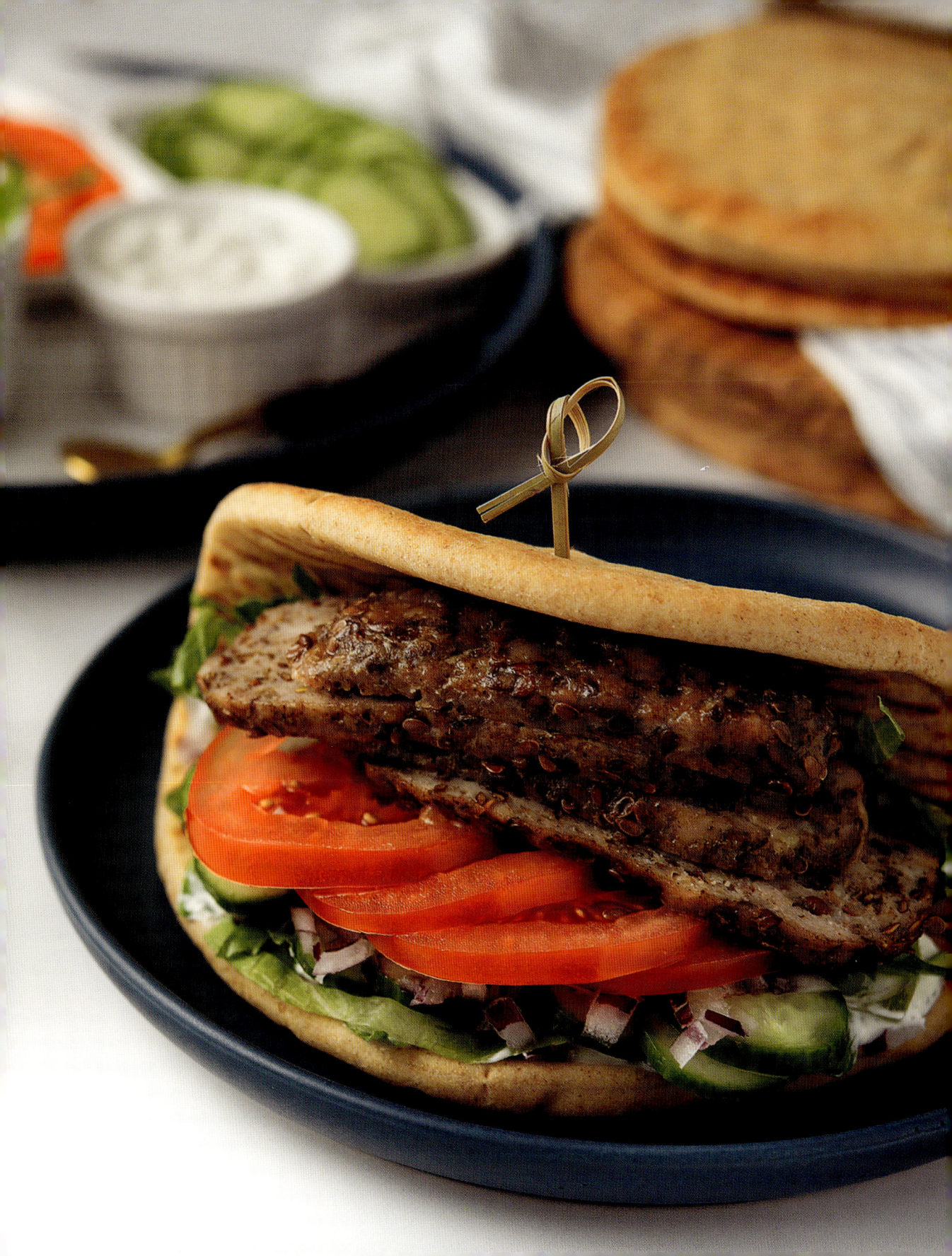

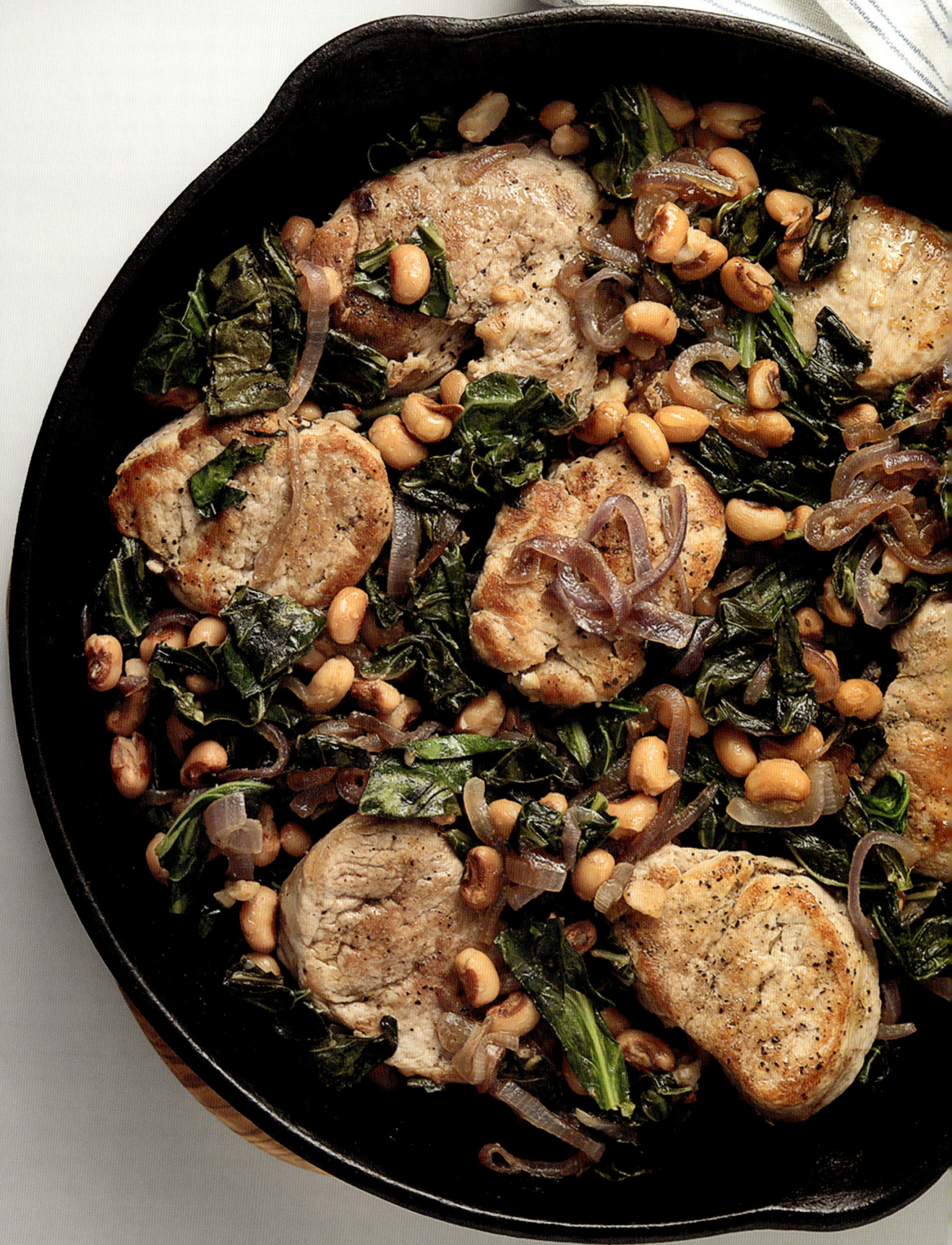

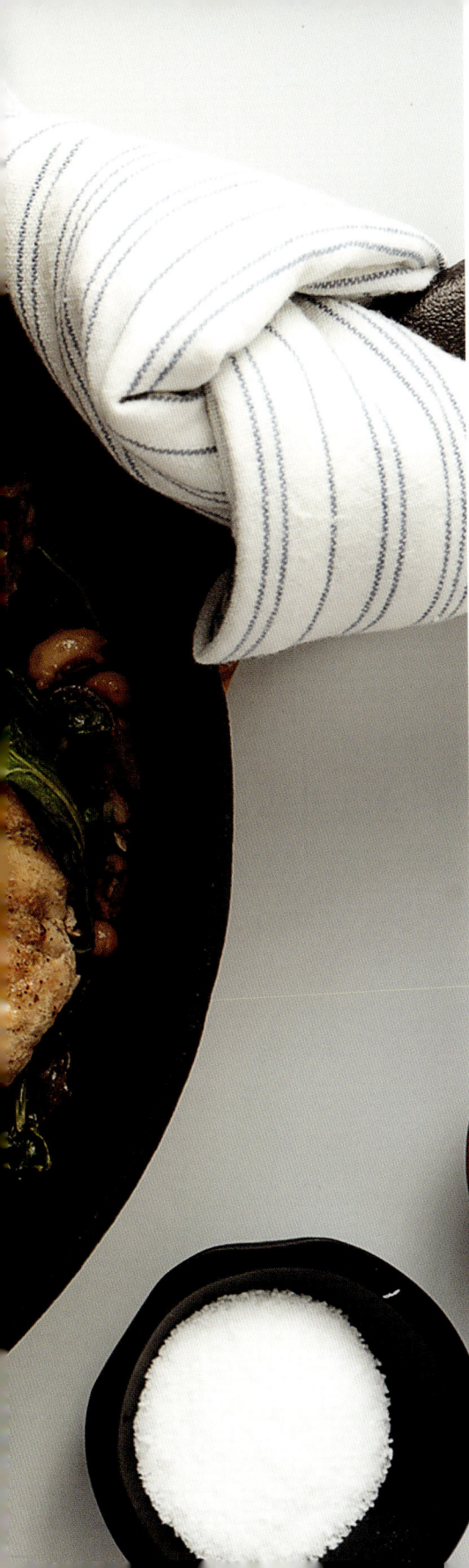

CHAPTER 5

30 Dinners in 30 Minutes

Weeknight meals need to be fast while still helping you achieve your nutrient needs to lower cholesterol. The dinner meals in this chapter were designed to help you squeeze in a home-cooked meal during a busy weeknight without sacrificing on flavor. While they can all be made in about 30 minutes or less, many can either be entirely made in advance or you can prepare components in advance to make these meals come together even quicker.

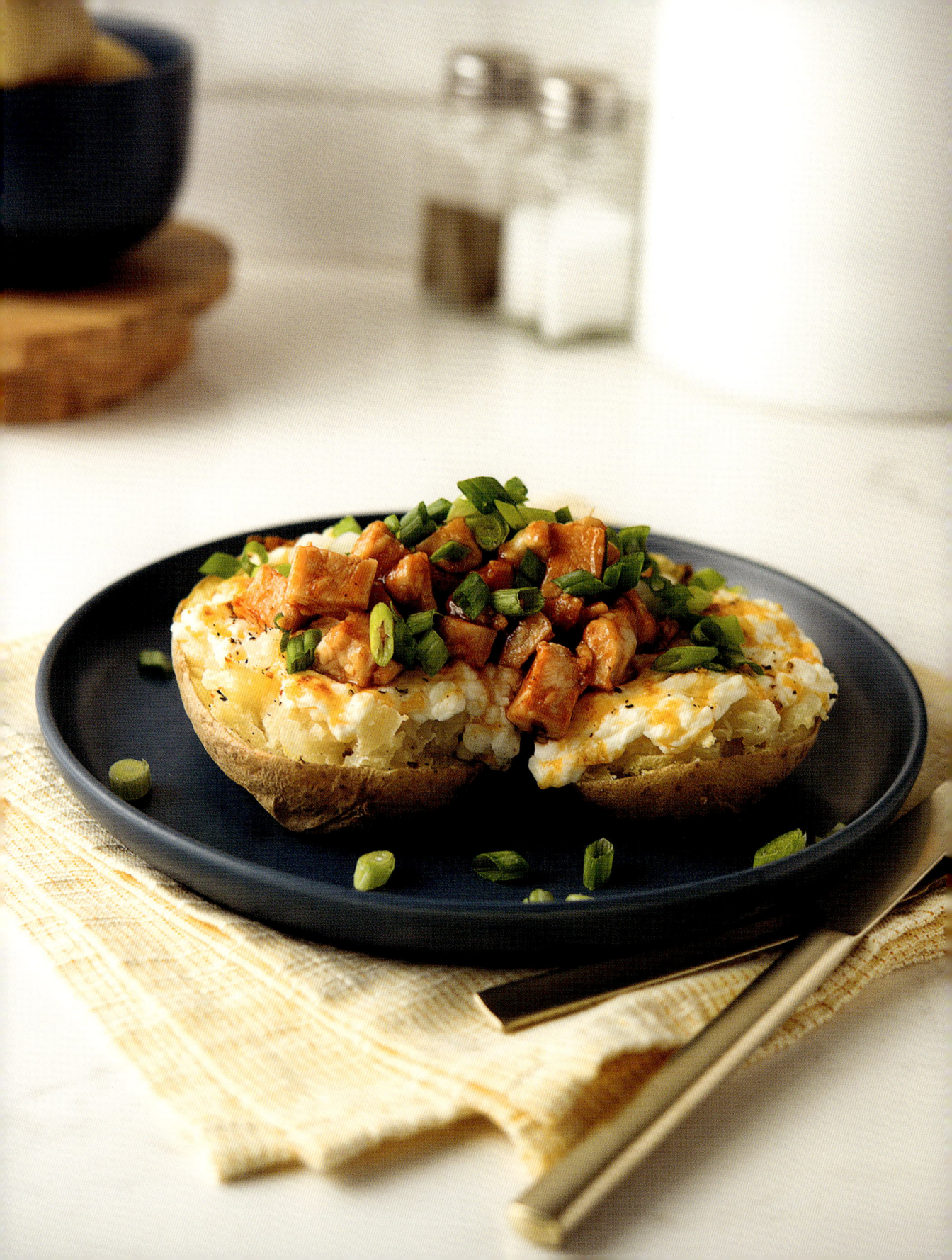

LOADED BAKED POTATO

A loaded baked potato might seem like something that should be off-limits when lowering your cholesterol, but this version swaps high-saturated-fat sour cream and butter for low-fat, protein-packed cottage cheese. The protein from the cottage cheese plus the fiber from the potato make this a comforting, filling, heart-healthy meal.

■ YIELD:
1 POTATO

■ PREP TIME:
5 MINUTES

■ COOK TIME:
15 MINUTES

1 russet potato

½ cup (115 g) low-fat cottage cheese

2 tablespoons (15 g) shredded sharp cheddar

1 cup (156 g) fresh or frozen broccoli

1 green onion, both green and white parts

Salt and pepper to taste

Wash and dry your potato. Poke it with a fork 4 to 6 times. Microwave on high for 6 minutes, then flip the potato (using an oven mitt). Microwave for 4 more minutes. Allow to sit in the microwave for 3 to 5 minutes before handling, then remove and set aside to cool slightly.

While the potato is cooking, mix together cottage cheese and shredded cheese. When the potato is done and cooling, add broccoli to microwave-safe dish and cook for 90 seconds on high.

When potato is cool enough to be handled, cut it in half and smash both sides using a fork until the flesh is flattened within the skin. Add broccoli to the top of the potato. Pour cheese mixture over the top. Microwave for 1 minute or pop it under the broiler to make it bubbly and crispy! Top with green onions and salt and pepper to taste.

NOTES

- Potatoes are actually a very healthy food. A medium potato contains about 40 percent of your daily requirement for potassium, an important nutrient for maintaining healthy blood pressure levels. It also has 7 grams of dietary fiber.

- Optional: Top with 2 pieces of crumbled turkey bacon or 2 ounces of chicken breast tossed in 1 tablespoon (15 g) barbecue sauce.

NUTRITIONAL ANALYSIS

SERVING SIZE: 1 baked potato

PER POTATO: 369 calories; 6 g fat; 4 g saturated fat; 27 g protein; 52 g carbohydrates; 7 g dietary fiber

OAT-CRUSTED CHICKEN THIGHS

Finding creative uses for oats is one of my favorite cooking experiments. This recipe was developed out of a desire to improve the fiber content of chicken tenders, and a delicious way to eat oats was born! These thighs taste great on a sandwich, on top of a salad, or eaten as a finger food with other dippable sides.

YIELD:
4 SERVINGS

PREP TIME:
10 MINUTES

COOK TIME:
15 MINUTES

¾ cup (60 g) rolled oats

2 tablespoons (28 ml) olive oil

1 teaspoon chili powder

1 teaspoon garlic powder

½ teaspoon salt

½ teaspoon ground black pepper

½ teaspoon ground cumin

2 egg whites

4 boneless, skinless chicken thighs, about 1 pound (455 g)

Put out 2 bowls for dredging the chicken. In one bowl, add oats, oil, and spices. Mix until the oats are thoroughly coated in the oil and spices. In the other bowl, add egg whites and whisk with a fork.

Pat chicken thighs dry with a paper towel. Use one hand to dip each chicken thigh in the egg white mixture, turning so both sides get coated, then place them in the oat mixture. Use the other hand to coat the chicken thighs with the oat mixture on both sides. Place in the bottom of the air fryer.

Air-fry the chicken thighs on 400°F (200°C) for 15 minutes until they reach an internal temperature of 165°F (74°C). If you don't have an air fryer, you can also make these in the oven. Place a wire baking rack onto a baking sheet to allow air to circulate around the chicken to crisp the oats. Spray the wire rack with nonstick spray and add chicken thighs on top. Bake in a preheated oven at 400°F (200°C or gas mark 6) for 18 to 20 minutes or until the internal temperature reaches 165°F (74°C).

There are many serving possibilities with these chicken thighs. You can add them to whole wheat bread for a "fried" chicken sandwich, slice them and add them on top of a salad, or cut them into cubes and serve like chicken nuggets with raw carrots, bell peppers, and sweet potato fries.

NUTRITIONAL ANALYSIS

SERVING SIZE: 1 chicken thigh

PER THIGH: 235 calories; 191 g fat; 2 g saturated fat; 21 g protein; 14 g carbohydrates; 2 g dietary fiber

NOTE

Looking for spicy chicken? Add ¼ teaspoon cayenne powder or 2 tablespoons (30 ml) hot sauce to the egg whites.

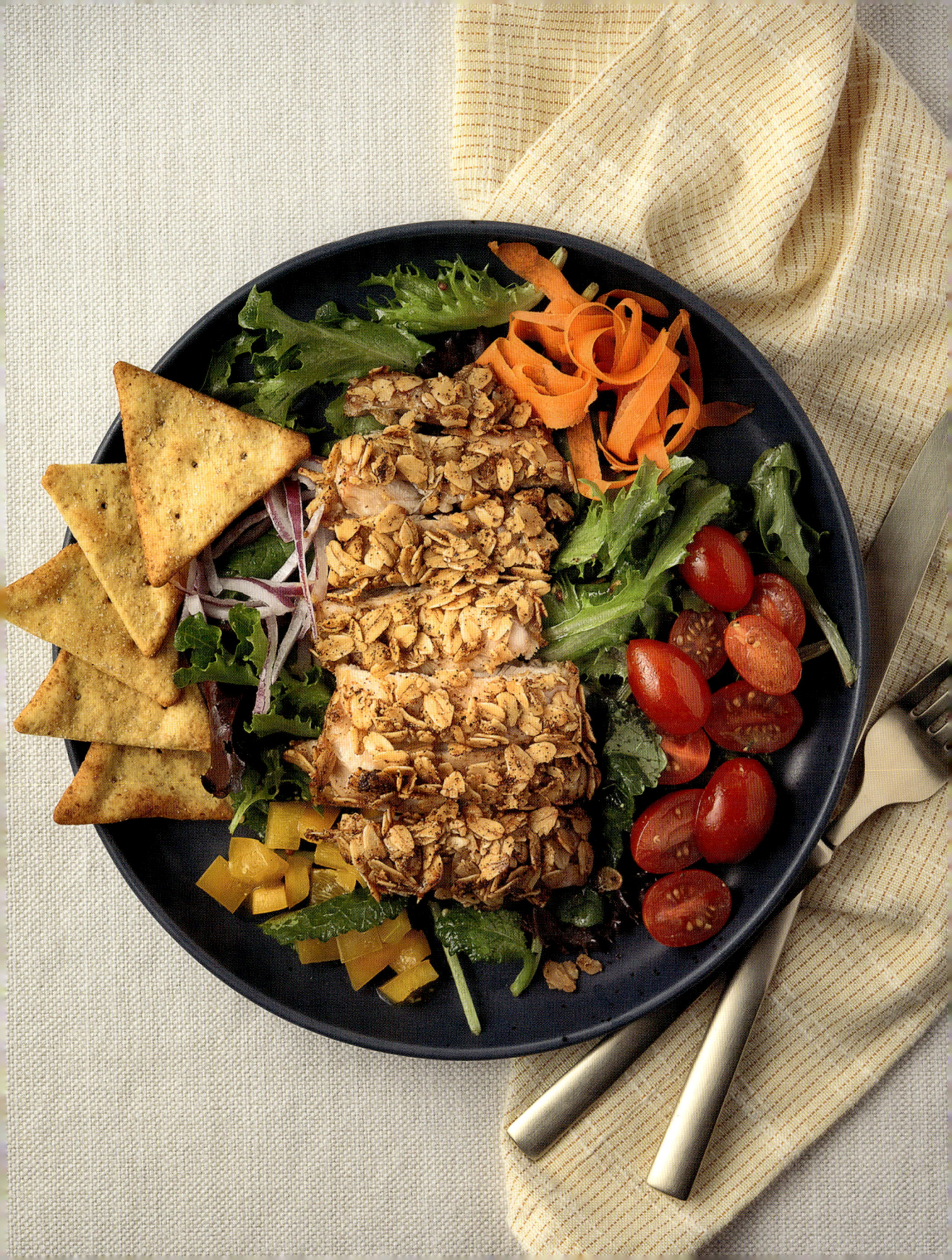

ONION AND ARTICHOKE BLENDED PASTA

■ **YIELD:**
3 SERVINGS

■ **PREP TIME:**
5 MINUTES

■ **COOK TIME:**
25 MINUTES

Blending cooked vegetables into a veggie-packed sauce is one of my favorite ways to spice up pasta night. Caramelized onions are the star of the show in this recipe. If you've never made caramelized onions, they are a labor of love. They take time, patience, and a lot of stirring over low heat to achieve without burning. It pays off in this decadent-tasting—but still heart-healthy—dish.

2 tablespoons (30 ml) olive oil

2 large onions, thinly sliced

1 teaspoon salt

¼ teaspoon ground black pepper

1 teaspoon dried thyme

Water or broth, as needed

3 garlic cloves, minced

1 box bean-based pasta, like Banza

1 cup (235 ml) reserved pasta cooking water, divided

½ cup (50 g) grated Parmesan cheese, plus 2 tablespoons (10 g) for garnish, divided

1 (14-ounce [397 g]) can artichoke hearts, drained

3 cups (90 g) fresh spinach

Add olive oil, onions, salt, pepper, and thyme to a large skillet over medium-low heat. Sauté the onions, stirring frequently, until the onions are caramelized, about 20 to 25 minutes. The onions will lose at least 50 percent of their volume and turn a nice golden brown color. If you find they are sticking to the pan, add a splash of water or broth. Add garlic in the final 3 minutes of cooking.

While the onions are caramelizing, bring pasta water to a boil and cook pasta according to package instructions. Reserve 1 cup (235 ml) pasta water to use in the sauce. Drain pasta and set aside.

When onions are done, add to a food processor with ¾ cup (175 ml) reserved pasta water and Parmesan cheese. Blend on high until a cohesive sauce forms. Next, add drained artichoke hearts and spinach and pulse 3 to 4 times. The veggies should be a little chunky, not completely blended into the sauce.

Add the sauce and remaining ¼ cup (60 ml) pasta water back to the pan. Turn the heat to medium-low and gently stir for 3 minutes. Add the pasta and stir to combine. Serve in a shallow bowl and top with 1½ teaspoons of Parmesan cheese for garnish.

NOTE

Caramelizing the onions will likely take longer than you think. I've built 20 to 25 minutes into this recipe just to get the right level of browning. Be patient! If you feel that you need more oil in the process, add a splash of chicken or vegetable broth every few minutes to keep the onions from sticking.

NUTRITIONAL ANALYSIS

SERVING SIZE: 2 cups (about 300 g) pasta

PER SERVING: 405 calories; 9 g fat; 3 g saturated fat; 23 g protein; 66 g carbohydrates; 10 g dietary fiber

CHICKEN AND BARLEY STIR-FRY

■ YIELD:
4 SERVINGS

■ PREP TIME:
10 MINUTES

■ COOK TIME:
15 MINUTES

Barley is an excellent substitute for rice in stir-fry recipes. Along with oats, barley is one of the most significant sources of beta-glucan, a particular type of soluble fiber that is especially effective at trapping and removing bile from the body, thereby lowering cholesterol levels. Paired with crunchy water chestnuts, tangy sauce, and lean chicken, this dish is a delightful meal.

1 cup (200 g) dried pearled barley

1 tablespoon (14 ml) olive or avocado oil

1 pound (455 g) ground chicken or turkey

1 pound (455 g) bok choy, sliced and rinsed

2 garlic cloves, minced

1 (8-ounce [225 g]) can sliced water chestnuts, drained

4 green onions, both green and white parts, sliced

¼ cup (60 ml) coconut aminos

2 tablespoons (28 ml) fresh-squeezed orange juice

1½ teaspoons fish sauce

1 teaspoon sesame oil

Prepare barley according to package instructions.

In a large sauté pan, add oil and ground meat. Cook over medium-high heat, using your spatula to break up the chicken or turkey, until completely cooked through, about 5 minutes. Add bok choy and continue cooking, stirring occasionally, until the bok choy begins to wilt. Then add in garlic, water chestnuts, and green onions. Stir and cook for 3 minutes.

Add in coconut aminos, orange juice, fish sauce, and sesame oil. Turn off the heat and stir to evenly coat all ingredients in the sauce. When barley is finished cooking, add it to the pan and mix to thoroughly coat in the sauce.

Plate and enjoy.

NOTES

- Coconut aminos is a soy sauce alternative that is slightly sweet in flavor and has considerably less sodium than soy sauce. It is a delicious and versatile addition to your kitchen pantry.

- Bok choy is a member of the cabbage family. It has many crevices that can lodge sediment. You should submerge the cut bok choy in a bowl of water and rinse it well before cooking. This will encourage the sediment to fall away into the bottom of the bowl and keep it out of your food.

- Any vegetables will work for this dish. Use what you have, but if it is not a leafy green, cook it in the olive oil for 5 minutes to soften before adding the chicken. Then proceed as instructed.

NUTRITIONAL ANALYSIS

SERVING SIZE: About 1½ cups (about 350 g) stir-fry

PER SERVING: 411 calories; 16 g fat; 4 g saturated fat; 27 g protein; 42 g carbohydrates; 8 g dietary fiber

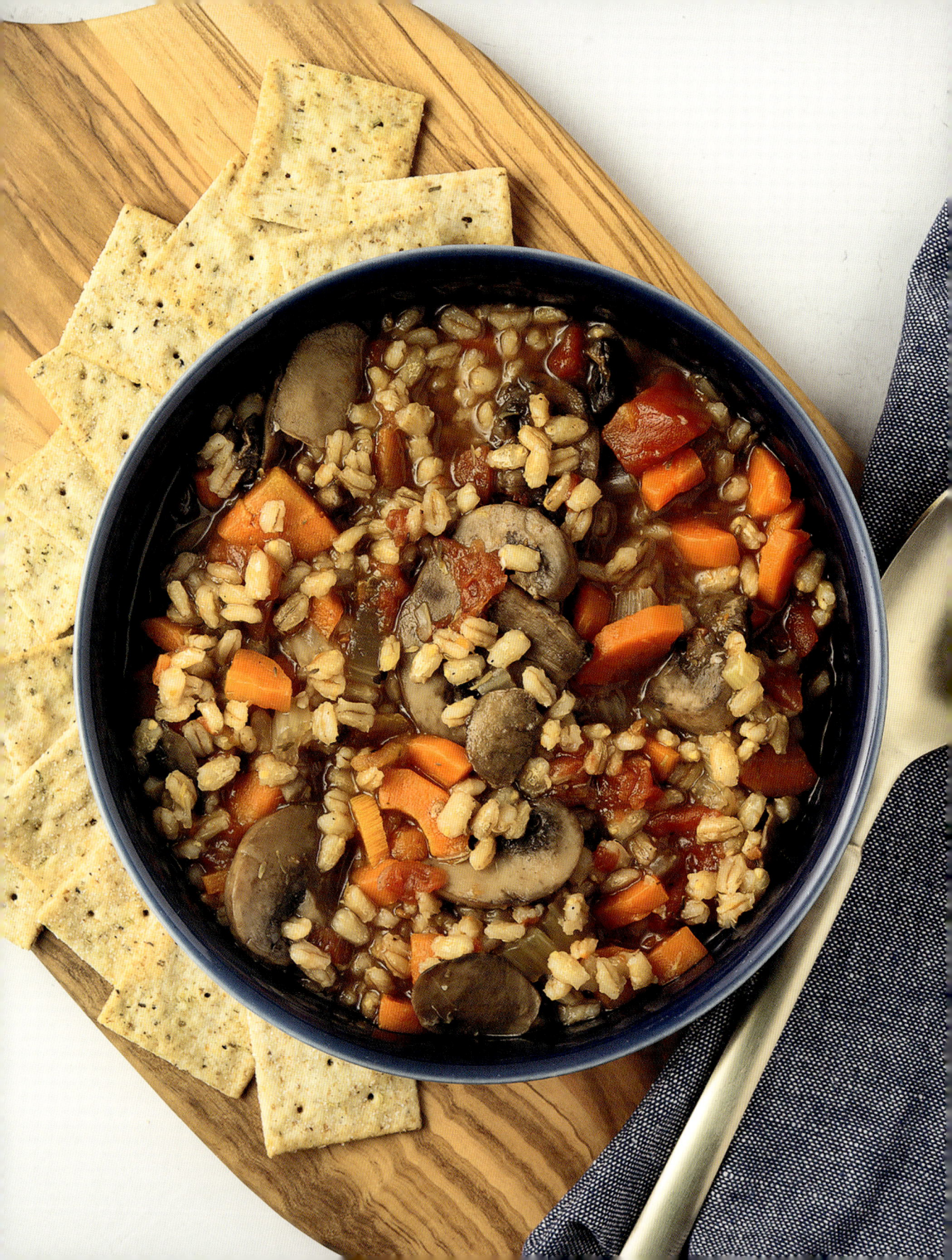

MUSHROOM BARLEY STEW

A twist on a classic beef and barley soup, this dish highlights mushrooms instead of beef. Cooked in an electric pressure cooker, it feels like a meal that has been simmering on the stove for hours rather than minutes. Complete with high-soluble-fiber barley, this stew is a delicious and filling addition to your day.

■ YIELD:
4 SERVINGS

■ PREP TIME:
5 MINUTES

■ COOK TIME:
25 MINUTES

3 carrots, diced

3 celery stalks, diced

1 large onion, diced

12 ounces (340 g) sliced mushrooms

3 garlic cloves, diced

1½ teaspoons salt

¼ teaspoon ground black pepper

1½ teaspoons dried thyme

1 cup (200 g) pearled barley

2 cups (475 ml) chicken or vegetable broth

1 (15.5-ounce [423 g]) can diced tomatoes

1 tablespoon (15 ml) olive oil, if making on stove

TO MAKE IN THE ELECTRIC PRESSURE COOKER

Combine all ingredients together in the electric pressure cooker. Cook under high pressure for 14 minutes, then do a quick release. Divide the soup between 4 bowls and serve.

TO MAKE ON THE STOVE

To make on the stove, this meal will take a bit longer. In the bottom of a soup pan over medium heat, add olive oil, carrots, celery, onion, and mushrooms. Sauté for 10 to 15 minutes until all of the vegetables are tender. Add garlic, salt, pepper, and thyme, and cook for 2 more minutes or until garlic is fragrant. Next, add barley, broth, and tomatoes. Cover and prepare according to barley package instructions.

NOTES

- This meal requires a bit of additional protein for most people. After calculating your protein needs from the equations in chapter 1, determine if you need additional protein for the day in this meal or if you can achieve your needs without it. If you do need more, you can add 3 ounces of animal protein, a side of low-fat cottage cheese, or a protein shake or yogurt bowl for dessert.

- You can also use this soup as a delicious first course to another protein-heavier option.

NUTRITIONAL ANALYSIS

SERVING SIZE: About 2 cups (about 375 g) soup

PER SERVING: 192 calories; 0 g fat; 0 g saturated fat; 8 g protein; 39 g carbohydrates; 9 g dietary fiber

SWEET AND SPICY CHICKPEAS

■ YIELD:
4 SERVINGS

■ PREP TIME:
10 MINUTES

■ COOK TIME:
20 MINUTES

This recipe is a flavorful and fiber-packed dinner that will leave you salivating and satisfied! The marriage of flavors and textures in this dish provides a comforting yet light combination or the chickpeas and rice. This is a true vegan dish that is delicious.

1 cup (158 g) brown rice

1½ teaspoons olive oil

1 large onion, sliced

2 bunches kale, chopped, about 8 cups (536 g), or 6 large handfuls greens

4 garlic cloves, minced

2 (15.5-ounce [423 g]) cans chickpeas, drained and rinsed

¼ cup (65 g) peanut butter or sunflower seed butter

2 tablespoons (32 g) miso paste

1½ tablespoons (25 ml) soy sauce

1 tablespoon (20 g) maple syrup

1 tablespoon (15 ml) rice vinegar

¼ cup (60 ml) water

½ teaspoon red pepper flakes

Cook brown rice according to package instructions and set aside.

While rice is cooking, add olive oil to a large skillet over medium-low heat. Add onions and sauté for 10 minutes or until tender and brown. Add in kale or greens and garlic and sauté for 5 to 7 minutes, until greens are completely wilted. Then add chickpeas and stir to combine.

In a small bowl, whisk together peanut butter or sunflower seed butter, miso paste, soy sauce, maple syrup, rice vinegar, water, and red pepper flakes. Pour over chickpea mixture and stir until it is completely coated in the sauce. Turn heat down to low and allow to bubble on the stove until the rice is ready, about 10 minutes. Stir frequently.

To serve, add chickpea mixture to the bottom of a bowl and top with ½ cup (79 g) rice.

NUTRITIONAL ANALYSIS

SERVING SIZE: ½ cup (79 g) rice + 2 cups (about 200 g) chickpeas

PER SERVING: 519 calories; 16 g fat; 3 g saturated fat; 20 g protein; 76 g carbohydrates; 15 g dietary fiber

NOTE

In the summer months, eggplant is an excellent addition to this dish, if you are a fan. It is a good source of fiber and antioxidants (in the skin). It adds a nice consistency to the dish.

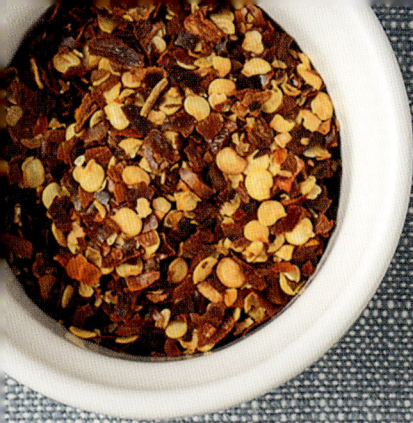

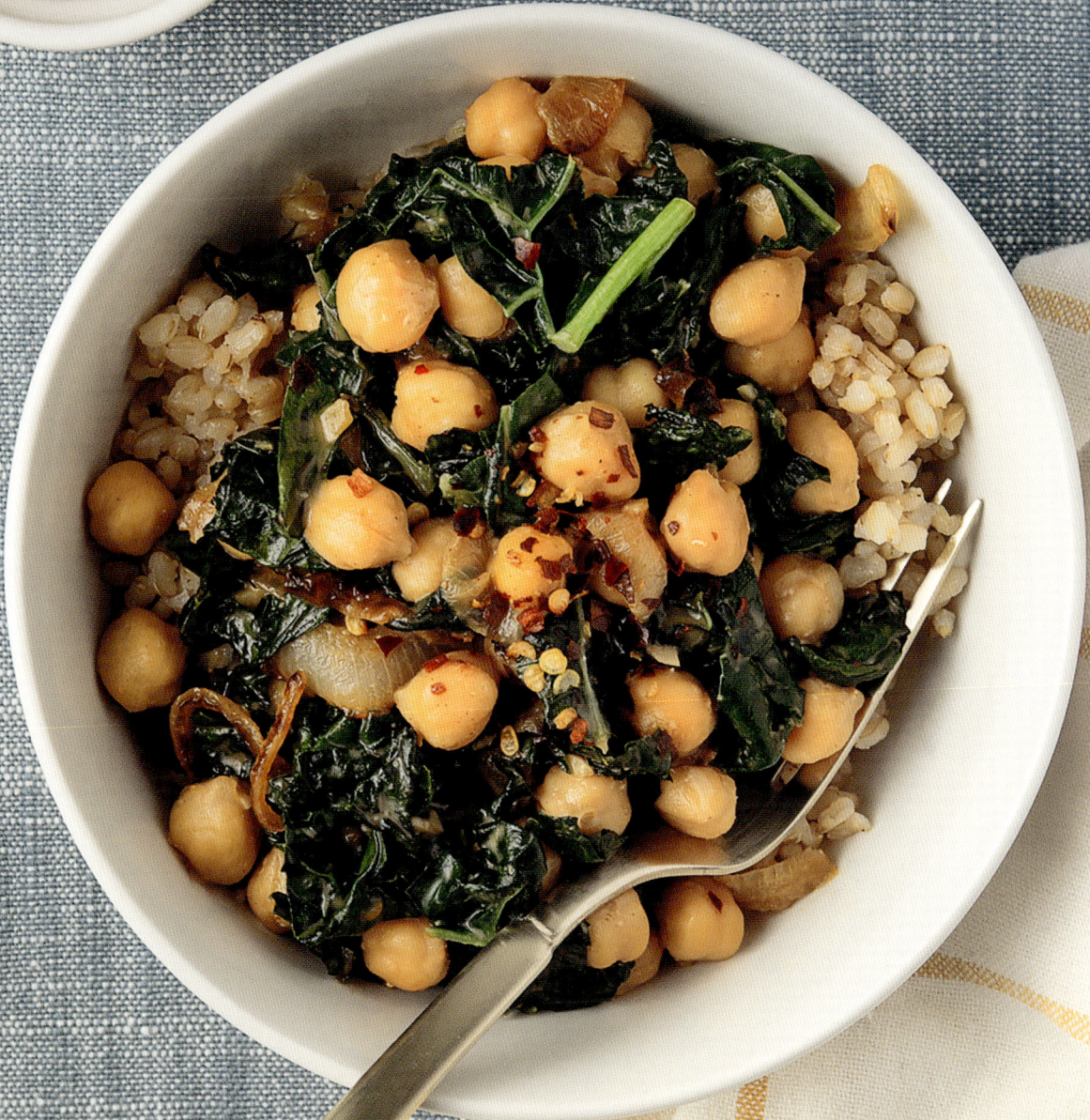

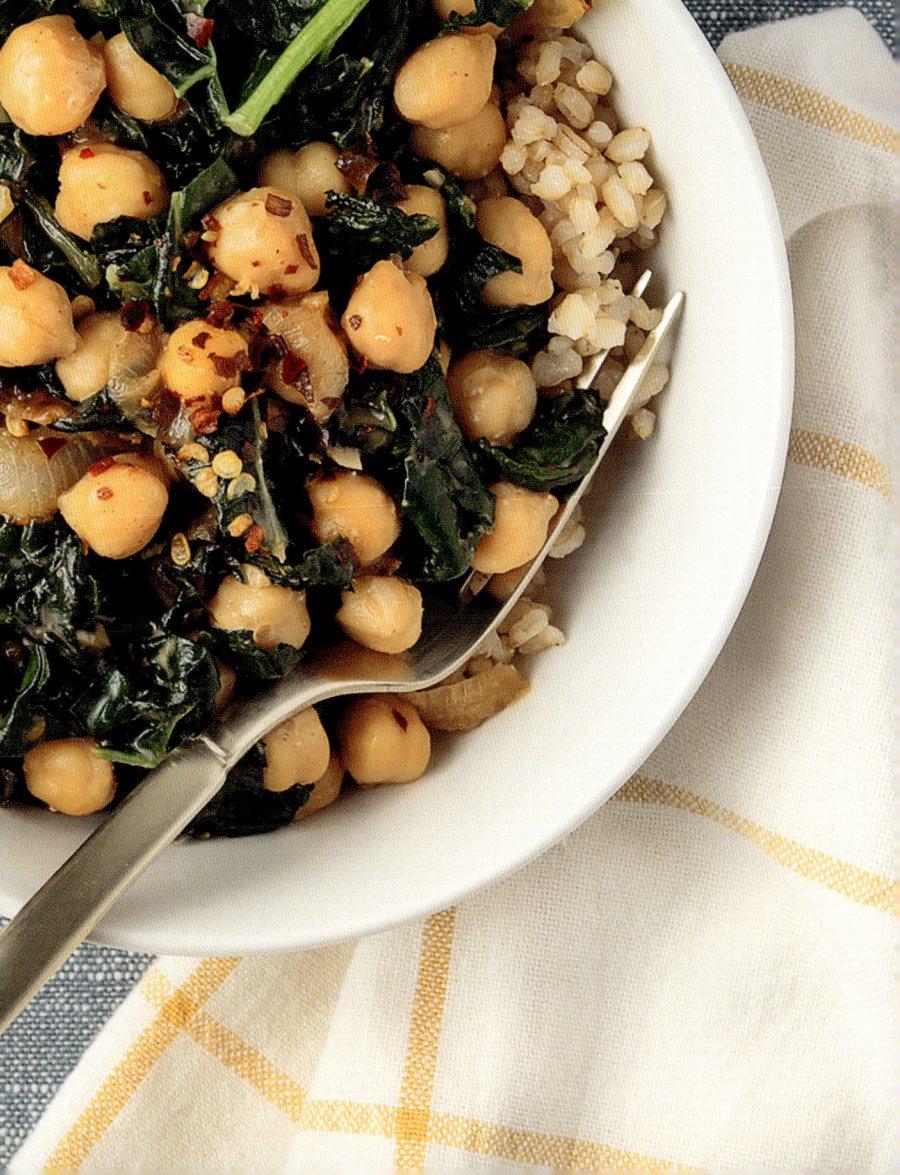

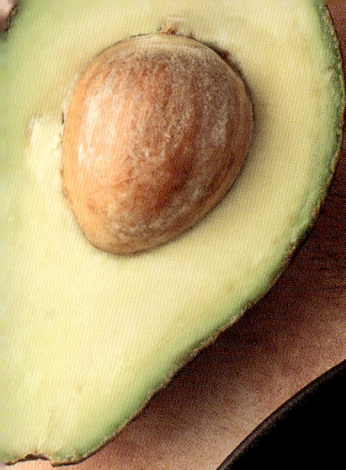

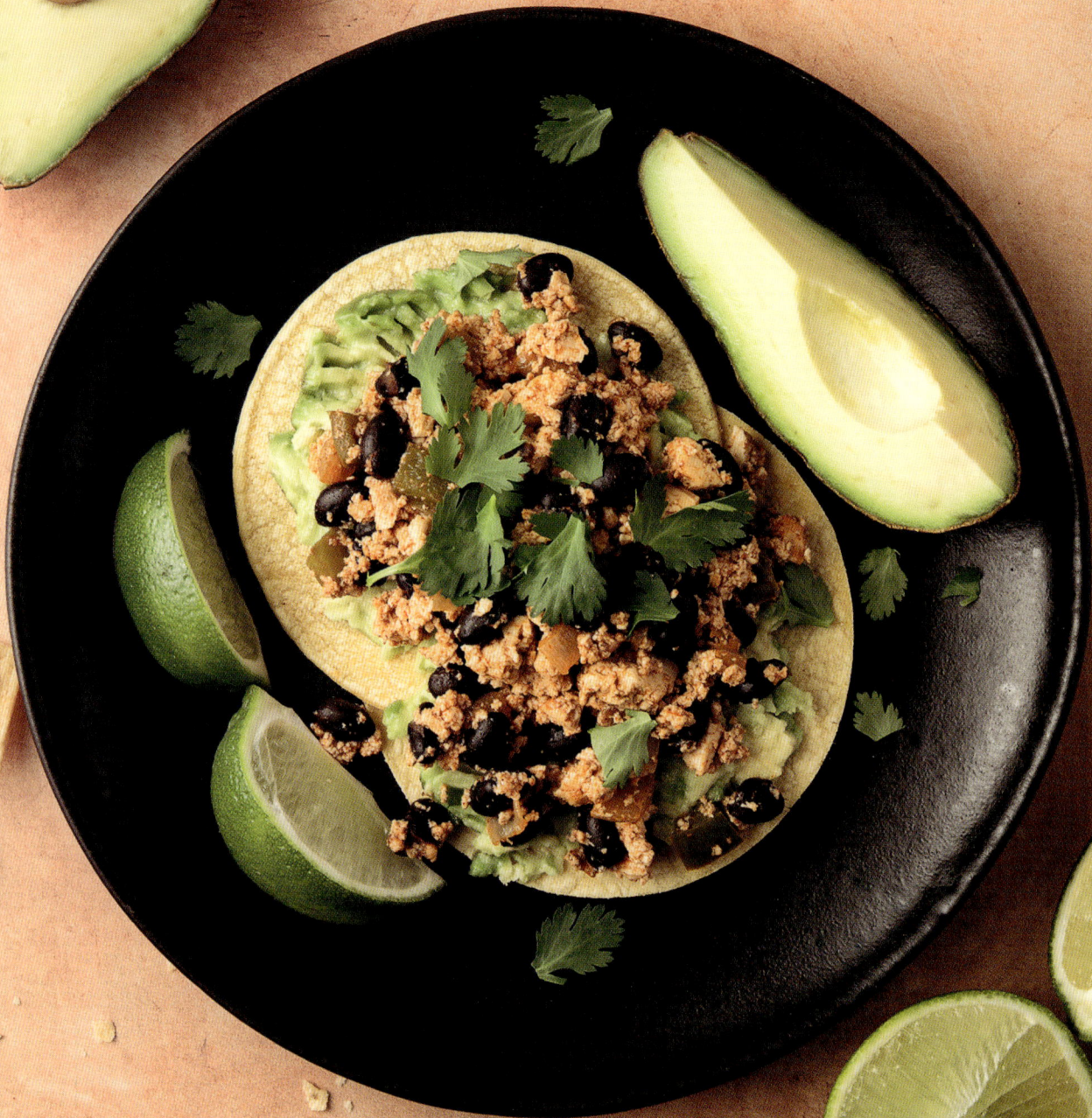

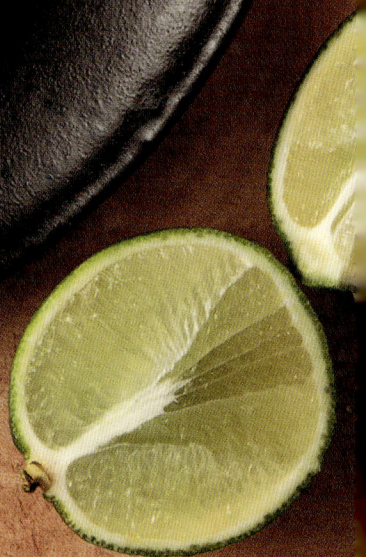

TOFU TACOS

This recipe was the first tofu dish I introduced to my husband many years ago. We had it over lettuce as a taco salad and he had no idea that it was tofu until after he'd cleaned his plate. Due to the strong flavors in the taco seasonings and the crumbled appearance, it is easy to mistake this dish for ground meat, making it the perfect gateway to tofu for you and your family. Plus, it has the added bonus of a quick cooking time!

■ **YIELD:**
4 SERVINGS

■ **PREP TIME:**
10 MINUTES

■ **COOK TIME:**
20 MINUTES

1 (15-ounce [420 g]) block extra-firm tofu

2 tablespoons (32 g) tomato paste

1 tablespoon (8 g) chili powder

1½ teaspoons soy sauce

1 tablespoon (15 ml) olive oil

1 large onion, diced

1 bell pepper, diced

2 teaspoons salt

1½ teaspoons garlic powder

1½ teaspoons ground cumin

1 (15.5-ounce [423 g]) can black beans, drained and rinsed

8 corn tortillas

1 avocado, quartered

Fresh cilantro for garnish, optional

In a large bowl, break up the tofu with your hands until it resembles ground meat. Add tomato paste, chili powder, and soy sauce, and mix. Set aside.

Add olive oil, onions, and peppers to a large skillet over medium-high heat and cook until tender, about 7 minutes. Add the tofu mixture, along with salt, garlic powder, and cumin. Cook for 4 to 5 minutes, then add black beans and stir to combine. Remove from heat.

Heat corn tortillas in the toaster, under the broiler, or in the microwave to soften them. Add 2 tortillas to each plate. Top each tortilla with one-eighth of the avocado and mash with a fork to spread over the tortilla. Add one-eighth of the mixture to each tortilla and garnish with cilantro, if using. Serve and enjoy!

NOTES

- No need to press this tofu! Pressing is a technique that is often used to remove excess liquid from the tofu. It can help to improve the texture when sautéing or baking tofu. In this recipe, the extra liquid will come out and evaporate. One less step to dinnertime!

- I love to add hot sauce to these tacos like I would for regular tacos. Bitchin' Sauce is a great brand for cholesterol-friendly and tasty dips and spreads.

- If serving this to your family, set up a taco bar and let them choose their own toppings.

NUTRITIONAL ANALYSIS

SERVING SIZE: 2 tacos

PER SERVING: 435 calories; 16 g fat; 2 g saturated fat; 21 g protein; 53 g carbohydrates; 17 g dietary fiber

TOFU AND CHICKPEA CURRY

Curry recipes tend to be high in saturated fat due to the use of coconut milk. Even though it is from a plant, coconut contains a higher percentage of saturated fat than butter! For this reason, the American Heart Association does not recommend coconut oil or coconut milk. Finding a creamy and delicious substitute was difficult, but this cashew and hemp sauce comes close!

■ **YIELD:**
4 SERVINGS

■ **PREP TIME:**
10 MINUTES

■ **COOK TIME:**
15 MINUTES

1 cup (158 g) brown rice

½ cup (68 g) cashews

¼ cup (30 g) hemp seeds

1⅓ cups (313 ml) boiling water

Nonstick cooking spray

1 white onion, thinly sliced

2 bell peppers, thinly sliced

3 handfuls fresh spinach

1 (15-ounce [420 g]) block firm tofu, cubed

1 (15.5-ounce [423 g]) can chickpeas, drained and rinsed

2 tablespoons (13 g) curry powder

½ teaspoon salt

1 tablespoon (20 g) honey

Fresh cilantro for garnish, optional

Cook brown rice according to package instructions.

Carefully add cashews, hemp seeds, and boiling water to a heat-safe jar. Allow to sit on the counter uncovered for 15 minutes. As the cashews and hemp seeds sit in the hot water, they will begin to soften and become easier to blend into a creamy sauce that we will use in place of coconut in our sauce.

Spray a large sauté pan with nonstick cooking spray and heat over medium-high heat. Sauté onion and pepper until tender, about 8 to 10 minutes. Then add in spinach, cubed tofu, and chickpeas. Reduce heat and stir occasionally while making sauce.

Add cashew mixture to a blender along with curry powder, salt, and honey. Blend on high for 30 to 60 seconds until a smooth, creamy sauce has formed. Add half of the sauce to the tofu pan and stir to combine. Add another one-quarter of the remaining sauce and stir. If your preferred level of sauciness has been achieved, reserve the remaining sauce. If you prefer a creamier sauce, add the rest of the mixture.

To serve, plate ½ cup (79 g) cooked brown rice. Serve curry on top. Garnish with cilantro, if using.

NUTRITIONAL ANALYSIS

SERVING SIZE: ½ cup (79 g) rice + 1 cup (about 256 g) curry

PER SERVING: 477 calories; 22 g fat; 5 g saturated fat; 20 g protein; 52 g carbohydrates; 7 g dietary fiber

MOROCCAN SPICED STUFFED PEPPERS

■ YIELD:
4 SERVINGS

■ PREP TIME:
5 MINUTES

■ COOK TIME:
25 MINUTES

This Moroccan spin on stuffed peppers makes a nice change from the typical flavor profile of these kinds of recipes. Made with warming spices, the hearty filling is loaded with dietary fiber and protein, while the raisins and nuts in the mix add sweetness and crunch.

1 cup (184 g) quinoa

4 bell peppers, any color

¼ cup (60 ml) water

1 tablespoon (15 ml) olive oil

1 large onion, diced

½ pound (225 g) ground chicken or turkey

2 garlic cloves, minced

1½ teaspoons allspice

½ teaspoon ground cinnamon

¾ teaspoon salt

1 cup (198 g) cooked lentils

⅓ cup (50 g) raisins

¼ cup (28 g) slivered almonds or walnuts

1 cup (180 g) frozen spinach or 4 cups (120 g) fresh spinach

¼ cup (60 ml) chicken or vegetable broth

2 tablespoons (3 g) chopped parsley

Preheat oven to 350°F (180°C or gas mark 4). Place a rack in the middle of the oven.

Prepare quinoa according to package instructions.

Halve the bell peppers. Remove the seeds and inner membrane. Lightly score the back of each pepper, making an X gently through the skin. Place open side down in a 9 × 13-inch (23 × 33 cm) baking dish with water. Place in the oven while the rest of the ingredients are cooking, about 15 minutes.

Add olive oil and onions to a large sauté pan over medium heat. Sauté until onions are tender, about 6 minutes, then add ground chicken or turkey. Break up the meat with your spatula so that it resembles ground meat. Add garlic, allspice, cinnamon, and salt. Cook until meat is completely cooked through, about 8 minutes.

When quinoa is finished cooking, add it to the sauté pan, along with lentils, raisins, nuts, spinach, and broth. Cook, stirring to combine, until the spinach is wilted, approximately 5 minutes. Remove the peppers from the oven and evenly divide the mixture between the 8 pepper halves. Place back in the oven for 10 minutes or until peppers are tender. Remove from the oven and sprinkle with parsley.

NOTES

- This recipe is a great way to use up cooked grains. Barley or white or brown rice would also taste great in place of the quinoa.

- Did you know that quinoa is actually a seed, not a grain? It's considered a pseudocereal because it is used similarly to other grains but is classified differently. This is one reason why the protein content of quinoa (8 grams per 1 cup [185 g]) is double the amount of protein in other grains.

NUTRITIONAL ANALYSIS

SERVING SIZE: 2 pepper halves

PER SERVING: 418 calories; 19 g fat; 4 g saturated fat; 25 g protein; 43 g carbohydrates; 10 g dietary fiber

FLANK STEAK FAJITAS

Flank steak is another leaner cut of beef. It comes from the underbelly of the cow, the equivalent of their ab muscles. This muscle gets worked continuously, which makes it have less marbling, or fat, throughout. When you want red meat, flank steak is a good option to have.

■ **YIELD:**
4 SERVINGS

■ **PREP TIME:**
10 MINUTES

■ **COOK TIME:**
15 MINUTES

1 pound (455 g) flank steak

Juice of 1 lime

2 garlic cloves, minced

1 teaspoon plus ¾ teaspoon salt, divided

2 teaspoons ground cumin

1 tablespoon (15 ml) plus 1 teaspoon olive or avocado oil, divided

1 yellow bell pepper, thinly sliced

1 red bell pepper, thinly sliced

1 orange bell pepper, thinly sliced

1 large onion, thinly sliced

1 tablespoon (8 g) chili powder

¼ teaspoon ground black pepper

8 corn tortillas

Fresh cilantro for garnish, optional

Thinly slice the steak and add to a shallow bowl. Add lime juice, garlic, 1 teaspoon salt, cumin, and 1 teaspoon olive or avocado oil. Toss and set aside.

Heat remaining 1 tablespoon (15 ml) olive or avocado oil in large skillet over medium-high heat. Add peppers, onions, chili pepper, remaining ¾ teaspoon salt, and black pepper. Cook for 7 to 8 minutes, stirring frequently, until vegetables are soft. Remove veggies from the pan and add in steak. Cook for 3 to 4 minutes on one side, then flip and cook for an additional 2 to 3 minutes until cooked thoroughly. Add back in peppers and onions.

To serve, portion one-eighth of the fajita mixture onto a corn tortilla. Top with fresh cilantro, if desired.

NUTRITIONAL ANALYSIS

SERVING SIZE: 2 fajitas

PER SERVING: 362 calories; 15 g fat; 5 g saturated fat; 27 g protein; 29 g carbohydrates; 5 g dietary fiber

NOTE

To bean or not to bean? I am usually a big fan of adding beans to dishes, but when eating beef, I don't always recommend it. Beef is a significant source of dietary iron for most Americans. Fiber, especially from high-fiber foods like beans, can bind to iron and prevent its absorption. This is especially important for children, premenopausal women, and pregnant women, as their daily iron needs are very high (11 mg, 18 mg, and 28 mg, respectively). Iron deficiency is the most common micronutrient deficiency in the United States because of these groups. In order to maximize iron absorption, I don't recommend eating beans with beef for these groups. Men and postmenopausal women have much lower iron needs (8 mg and 9 mg, respectively) that are easier to achieve. If you fall into one of those two groups, feel free to add beans to dishes with beef for the added fiber!

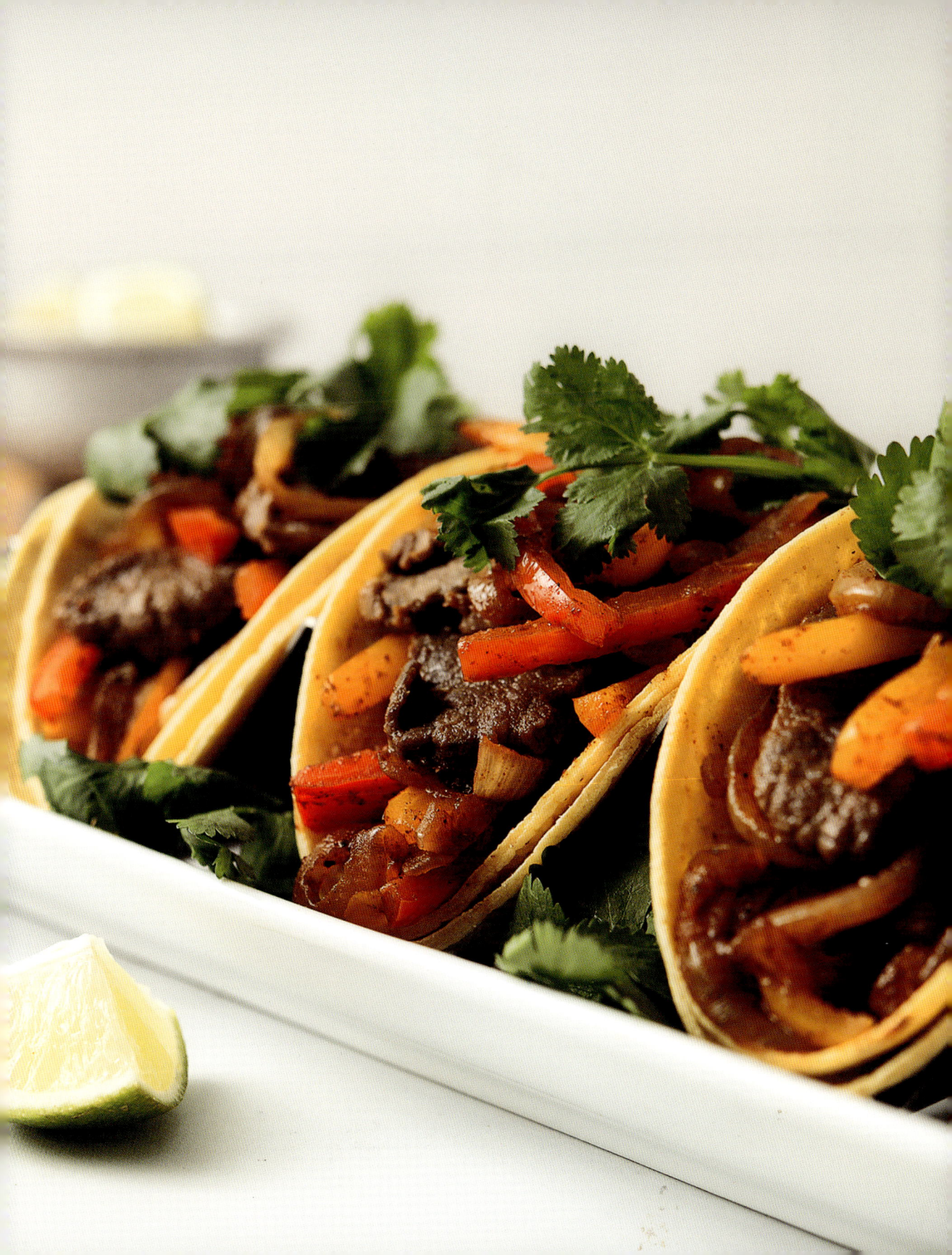

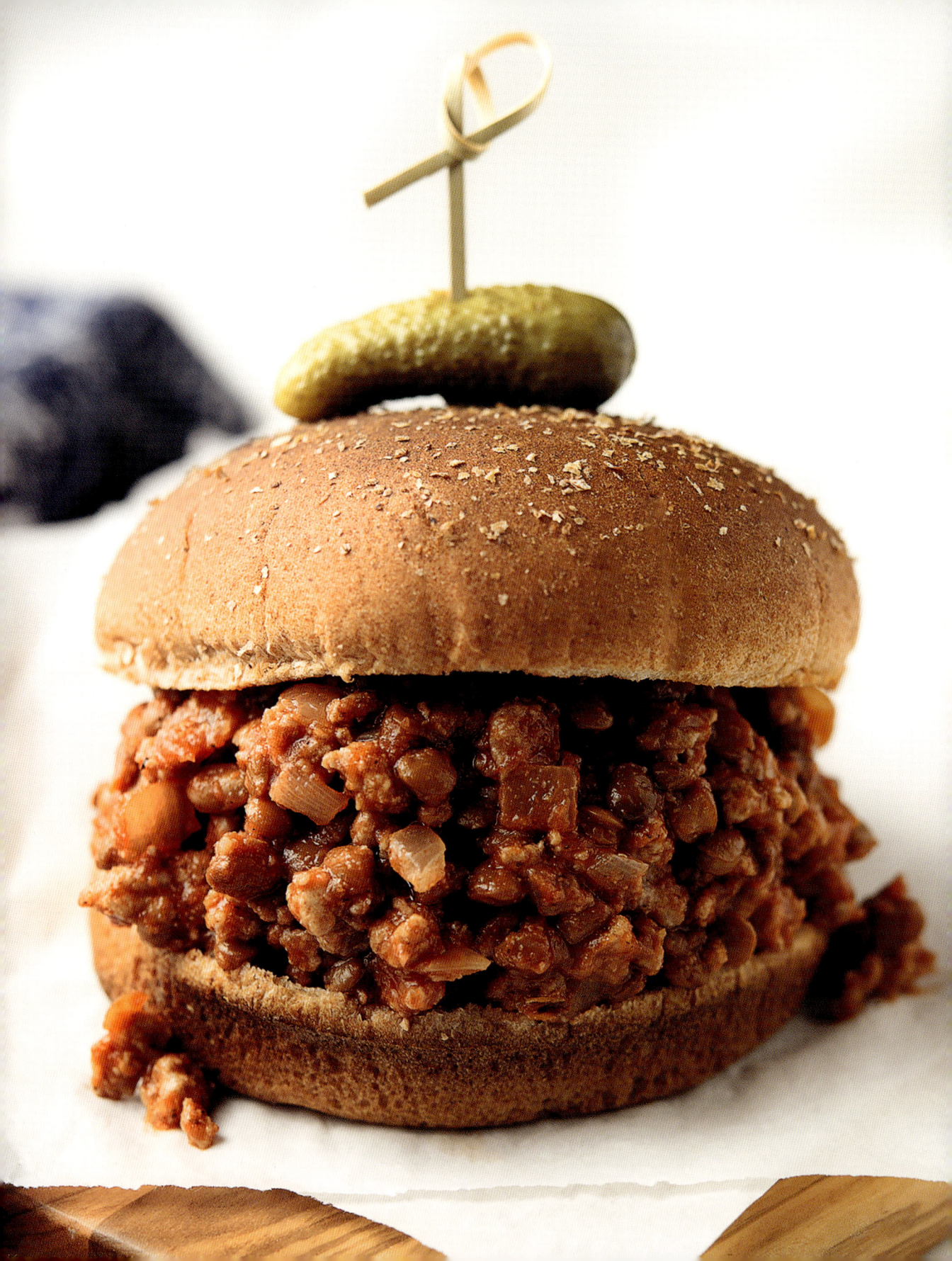

SLOPPY JOES

This is a childhood favorite that I still love to this day. The perfect balance of sweet and tangy, this sloppy joe recipe is packed with fiber and protein.

■ **YIELD:**
4 SERVINGS

■ **PREP TIME:**
5 MINUTES

■ **COOK TIME:**
20 MINUTES

1 tablespoon (15 ml) olive oil

1 large onion, diced

1 pound (455 g) ground turkey

1 teaspoon ground cumin

1 tablespoon (9 g) garlic powder

2 teaspoons salt

½ teaspoon ground black pepper

2½ tablespoons (36 ml) red wine vinegar

1 (6-ounce [168 g]) can tomato paste

¾ cup (175 ml) water, plus more as needed

1 (15-ounce [420 g]) can lentils, drained and rinsed

4 whole wheat buns

In a large skillet, heat olive oil over medium heat. Sauté onions, stirring often, until tender and beginning to brown, about 8 minutes. Add ground turkey and cook until browned, about 10 minutes.

Next, add cumin, garlic powder, salt, pepper, vinegar, and tomato paste. Fill the empty tomato paste can with water, stir to incorporate any leftover paste, and add to the pan. Bring back up to a low simmer. Add lentils and stir to combine. Turn down the heat and allow to simmer for 5 minutes. If it looks like it is drying out, add 1 tablespoon (15 ml) water at a time.

To serve, toast the buns and top with sloppy joe mixture. Remember, it will be sloppy! Expect some to fall off the sides.

NUTRITIONAL ANALYSIS

SERVING SIZE: 1 sandwich

PER SERVING: 526 calories; 16 g fat; 4 g saturated fat; 40 g protein; 58 g carbohydrates; 14 g dietary fiber

NOTE

The sweetness in this recipe comes from the tomato paste. Since tomato pastes can vary widely, if you feel the recipe needs more sweetness to balance the acidity of the vinegar, add 1 teaspoon sugar or maple syrup at a time, stir, and taste again until you reach the right balance. Aim to stay under 1 tablespoon (12 g) total, though.

MINESTRONE

Packed with hearty vegetables and beans, this classic minestrone soup is high in fiber and very filling. The tomato base is a good source of lycopene, an antioxidant that may help to protect against heart disease. This soup recipe feeds a crowd! I recommend freezing leftovers in single-serving containers for a quick, weeknight meal option.

■ **YIELD:**
6 SERVINGS

■ **PREP TIME:**
5 MINUTES

■ **COOK TIME:**
20 MINUTES

1 tablespoon (15 ml) olive oil

1 medium onion, diced

2 medium carrots, diced

2 celery stalks, diced

3 garlic cloves, minced

1 (32-ounce [950 ml]) carton vegetable broth

2 cups (475 ml) water

1 (28-ounce [785 g]) can crushed tomatoes

1 (15.5-ounce [423 g]) can kidney beans, drained and rinsed

1 (15.5-ounce [423 g]) can chickpeas, drained and rinsed

1½ cups (186 g) frozen green beans

1 tablespoon (4 g) Italian seasoning

2 bay leaves

1 bunch kale, chopped, about 4 cups (268 g)

¼ cup (65 g) pesto

Salt, to taste

Ground black pepper, to taste

Heat olive oil in a large pot over medium heat. Add onions, carrots, and celery, and sauté, stirring often, for 5 to 7 minutes, or until the onions are fragrant and translucent. Add garlic and cook for another 2 minutes. Add vegetable broth, water, tomatoes, kidney beans, chickpeas, green beans, Italian seasoning, and bay leaves. Mix everything together until well combined and bring the mixture to a boil.

Remove from heat, mix in kale and pesto, and allow the soup to cool for about 5 minutes.

Remove bay leaves. Season with salt and pepper to taste. Enjoy!

NUTRITIONAL ANALYSIS

SERVING SIZE: About 2 cups (about 350 g) minestrone

PER SERVING: 402 calories; 16 g fat; 1 g saturated fat; 17 g protein; 51 g carbohydrates; 14 g dietary fiber

NOTES

- Looking for more protein in this meal? Add 2 ounces (55 g) cooked chicken breast per serving for an additional 100 calories, 15 grams of protein, 4 grams of fat, 0 grams of saturated fat, and 0 grams of carbohydrates.

- One tablespoon (5 g) Parmesan cheese adds only 1 gram of saturated fat to this low–saturated fat recipe!

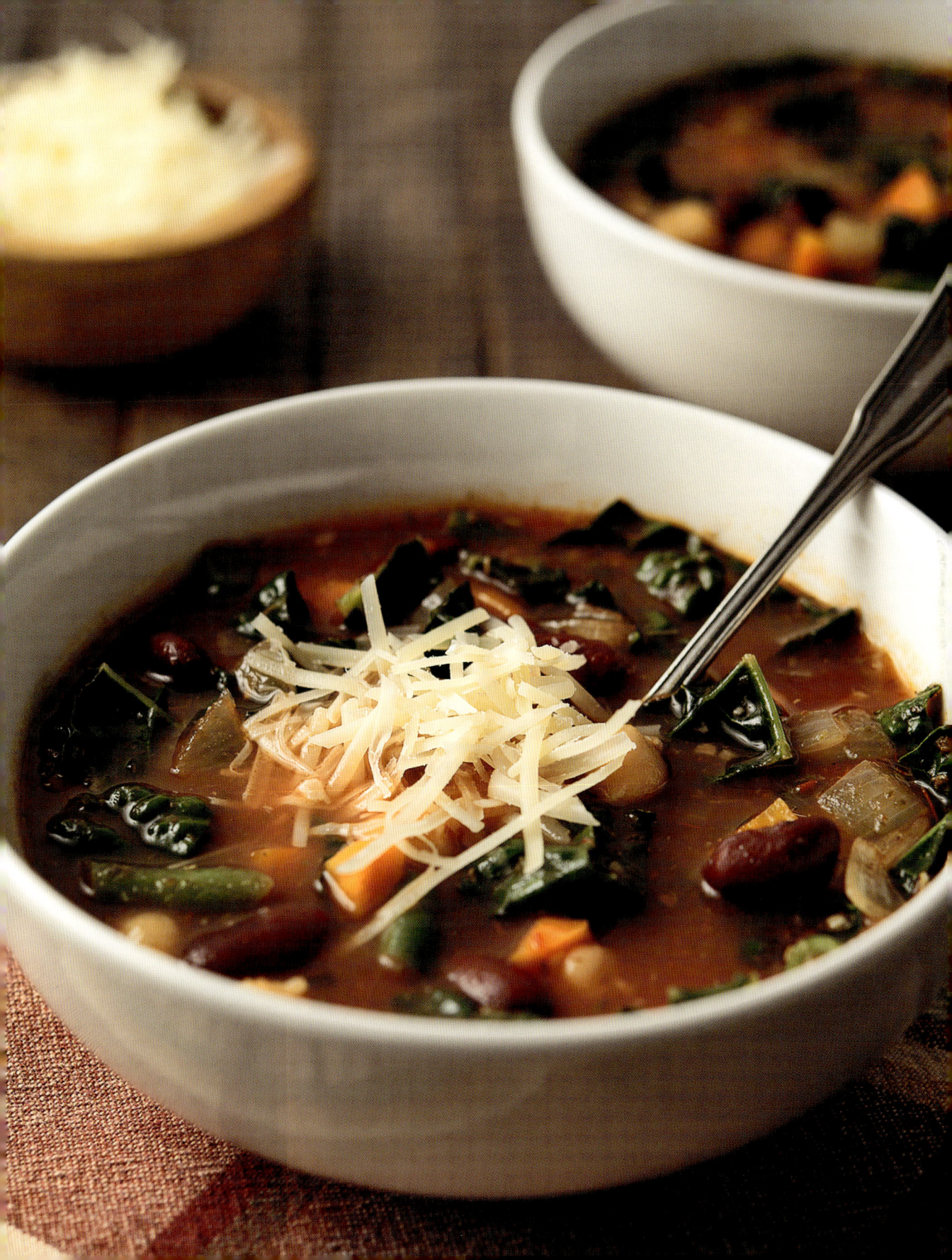

WEEKNIGHT BEEF STEW

■ YIELD:
4 SERVINGS

■ PREP TIME:
5 MINUTES

■ COOK TIME:
25 MINUTES

Stew cuts of beef, like shoulder or round roasts, are lower in saturated fat than more tender cuts like steaks or ground meat. Roasts typically come from large, heavily used muscles that have more connective tissue and thicker muscle fibers. Because of this, stews need to be cooked with a "low and slow" method to tenderize the meat and break down the connective tissue. Thank goodness for the electric pressure cooker, which gives us the same effect without the hours of cooking!

2 cups (260 g) prechopped mirepoix (onions, celery, carrots) (see Notes)

8 ounces (225 g) sliced mushrooms

1 (15-ounce [420 g]) can diced tomatoes

2 cups (475 ml) beef, chicken, or vegetable broth

1 pound (455 g) beef chuck, shoulder, or roast, cubed into ½-inch (1 cm) pieces

1 pound (455 g) yellow potatoes, quartered or cubed into ½-inch (1 cm) pieces

1 teaspoon salt

½ teaspoon ground black pepper

1 teaspoon garlic

1 teaspoon dried thyme

1 teaspoon dried rosemary

1 tablespoon (8 g) flour (white or wheat)

¼ cup (60 ml) water

1 cup (130 g) frozen green peas

NUTRITIONAL ANALYSIS

SERVING SIZE: About 1½ cups (about 500 g) stew

PER SERVING: 402 calories; 16 g fat; 1 g saturated fat; 17 g protein; 51 g carbohydrates; 14 g dietary fiber

Add mirepoix, mushrooms, diced tomatoes, broth, beef, potatoes, salt, black pepper, garlic, thyme, and rosemary to the electric pressure cooker. Stir to combine, then cook on high pressure for 20 minutes. When time expires, do a quick release. If you have time for natural release, allow it. It will help to further tenderize the meat.

Switch the electric pressure cooker to the sauté function. Mix flour and water together in a small bowl until dissolved. Stir into the stew and allow to bubble for 5 minutes. Select Cancel to turn off sauté, then add frozen peas. They will cook in the hot stew and help to cool it down to eat. Divide your stew between 4 bowls and enjoy!

NOTES

- Can't find precut veggies? Two cups (260 g) of the mix is roughly 1 large onion, 2 large carrots, and 3 celery stalks. Precut mirepoix is often available in the pre-prepared or packaged vegetable section at the store. You can also find this mix in the freezer section at some stores.

- If you don't have an electric pressure cooker, this recipe can be made on the stove. Sauté the vegetables until tender before adding the meat and browning on both sides. Then add tomatoes, broth, and seasonings. Bring to a boil, then reduce to a simmer for 1 to 1½ hours. Add a slurry to thicken the stew after the meat is tender, and add the peas at the end.

MACARONI AND CHEESE

Once again, blended cottage cheese turns a high-fat comfort food into a heart-friendly meal. It really is a versatile ingredient that lowers saturated fat and boosts protein with just one easy swap.

■ **YIELD:**
3 SERVINGS

■ **PREP TIME:**
5 MINUTES

■ **COOK TIME:**
15 MINUTES

- 1 (8-ounce [225 g]) box bean-based elbow noodle pasta, like Banza
- 2 cups (312 g) frozen broccoli
- ¾ cup (169 g) low-fat cottage cheese
- ½ cup (50 g) grated Parmesan cheese
- ½ cup (58 g) shredded sharp cheddar
- ½ cup (120 ml) reserved cooking liquid
- ½ teaspoon dried thyme
- ⅛ teaspoon ground black pepper

Bring a large pot of water to a boil and cook pasta according to package instructions. When pasta is roughly 2 minutes from being done, remove ½ cup (120 ml) starchy cooking water from the pan and reserve. Add frozen broccoli to the pasta pot and bring water back up to a boil.

In a food processor, add cottage cheese, Parmesan cheese, cheddar cheese, reserved starchy pasta water, thyme, and black pepper. Blend for 60 to 90 seconds or until a smooth, creamy sauce has formed.

Drain the pasta and broccoli and add back to the pot. Stir in the cheese mixture and heat over medium-low heat until cheese sauce thickens and coats the noodles and broccoli. Serve.

NOTES

- This macaroni and cheese tastes great if you have time to bake it in the oven to get a crispier topping. It also tastes even better the next day, in my opinion, so consider making enough for lunch the next day.

- The starchy cooking liquid helps to thicken the cheese sauce. Adding the water while it is still very hot also helps to melt the cheeses so they become creamy.

NUTRITIONAL ANALYSIS

SERVING SIZE: About 2½ cups (about 250 g) pasta

PER SERVING: 390 calories; 10 g fat; 3 g saturated fat; 27 g protein; 55 g carbohydrates; 8 g dietary fiber

PIZZA WITH ARTICHOKE, PESTO, AND MOZZARELLA

■ **YIELD:**
4 SERVINGS

■ **PREP TIME:**
10 MINUTES

■ **COOK TIME:**
12 MINUTES

Making pizza at home is the best way to continue enjoying this much-beloved food while lowering your cholesterol. When you make it at home, you can control the amount of cheese you add, thus controlling the saturated-fat content. The base recipe below features an artichoke and pesto sauce (with a fiber boost from the ground flaxseed) and mozzarella cheese. Feel free to personalize it with your own favorite toppings; just note this will affect the nutritional content.

- 1 pound (455 g) pizza dough, or one ball
- 1 (14-ounce [397 g]) can artichoke hearts, drained and squeezed to expel extra water
- 1 (6-ounce [168 g]) can tomato paste (see Notes)
- 1 tablespoon (15 ml) olive oil
- 1 tablespoon (15 g) pesto
- 1 teaspoon salt
- 1 teaspoon Italian seasoning
- 1 teaspoon garlic powder
- ¼ cup (28 g) ground flaxseed or flaxseed meal
- 1–2 tablespoons (15–28 ml) water, as needed
- 2 tablespoons (18 g) cornmeal or polenta
- 1 cup (115 g) shredded mozzarella cheese
- 4 cups (220 g) side salad of choice

Preheat oven to 425°F (220°C or gas mark 7) and place the rack in the center of the oven. Remove pizza dough from the refrigerator to allow to come to room temperature while preparing the sauce.

In a food processor or blender, combine drained artichoke hearts, tomato paste, olive oil, pesto, salt, Italian seasoning, garlic powder, and flaxseed. Blend on high until a cohesive paste forms, about 2 minutes. If paste is too thick, add 1 tablespoon (15 ml) water at a time until a spreadable paste forms. You may not need water, depending on how much liquid remains in the artichokes.

NUTRITIONAL ANALYSIS

SERVING SIZE: ¼ pizza

PER SERVING: 502 calories; 18 g fat; 4 g saturated fat; 22 g protein; 65 g carbohydrates; 5 g dietary fiber

NOTES

- Tomato paste matters! If you can, pick a highly concentrated paste that has a big tomato flavor.
- This sauce is relatively thick, so you will end up with a thick layer of sauce that will condense during cooking.

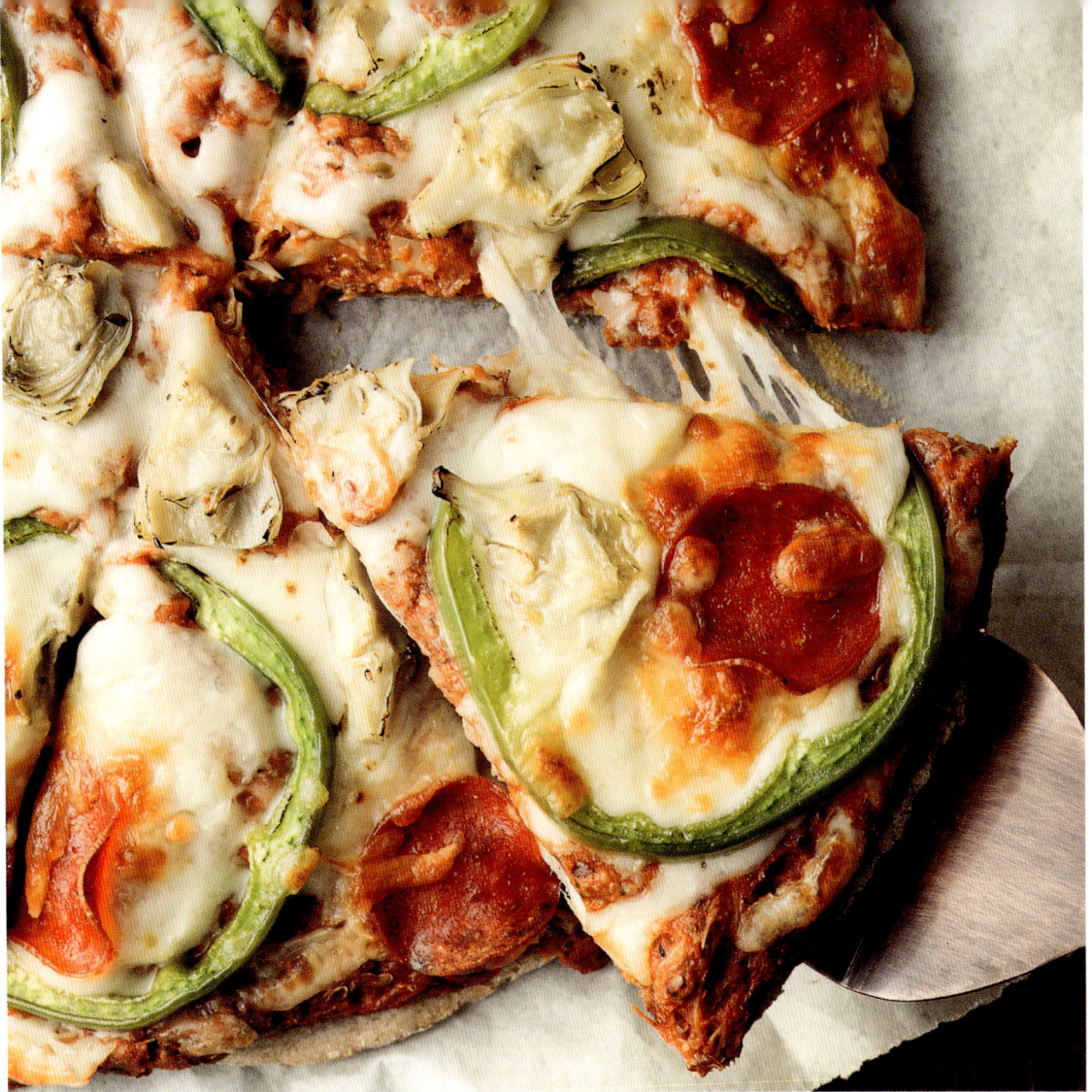

OPTIONAL EXTRA TOPPINGS

Mushrooms

Peppers

Onions

Spinach

Artichokes

Turkey pepperoni

Line a baking sheet with parchment paper and evenly scatter cornmeal or polenta on the parchment paper. Stretch the pizza dough into a large circle and lay on top. Evenly spread artichoke sauce on pizza (it will be a thick layer), then top with shredded mozzarella cheese and any additional toppings.

Bake for 12 minutes or until the center of the pizza is cooked through. Serve one-quarter of the pizza with 1 cup (55 g) side salad for added fiber.

PORK TENDERLOIN MEDALLIONS, BLACK-EYED PEAS, AND COLLARD GREENS

■ **YIELD:**
4 SERVINGS

■ **PREP TIME:**
15 MINUTES

■ **COOK TIME:**
15 MINUTES

Symbolizing good luck and prosperity, this is a classic meal served on New Year's Day in the South to set the tone for the year to come. While most cuts of pork are high in saturated fat, pork tenderloin is a leaner cut that is relatively low in saturated fat, making it a good option for lowering cholesterol levels while still enjoying foods you love.

FOR THE GREENS AND PEAS

2 bunches collard greens, trimmed and roughly chopped (see Note)

½ red onion, thinly sliced

1 tablespoon (15 ml) olive oil

¼ teaspoon salt

1 (15.5-ounce [423 g]) can black-eyed peas, drained and rinsed

1 tablespoon (15 ml) balsamic or apple cider vinegar

1 garlic clove, minced

TO MAKE THE GREENS AND PEAS

Add collard greens, red onion, olive oil, and salt to a large pan over medium-low heat. Cook, stirring frequently, until greens are very wilted and onion is soft, about 15 to 20 minutes. If you notice the greens or onion beginning to burn, turn down heat. When the greens and onion are very tender, add black-eyed peas, vinegar, and garlic. Allow to cook for 2 to 3 more minutes on low, or until pork is ready to serve.

NUTRITIONAL ANALYSIS

SERVING SIZE: ¾ cup (about 75 g) beans and greens mix + 2 medallions

PER SERVING: 347 calories; 11 g fat; 2 g saturated fat; 34 g protein; 29 g carbohydrates; 11 g dietary fiber

NOTE

To trim your collard greens, first cut out the tough middle stem. Fold each leaf in half and run your knife along the inside of the stem. When you open the green, you should see a long, thin triangle missing from the leaf and no visible stem.

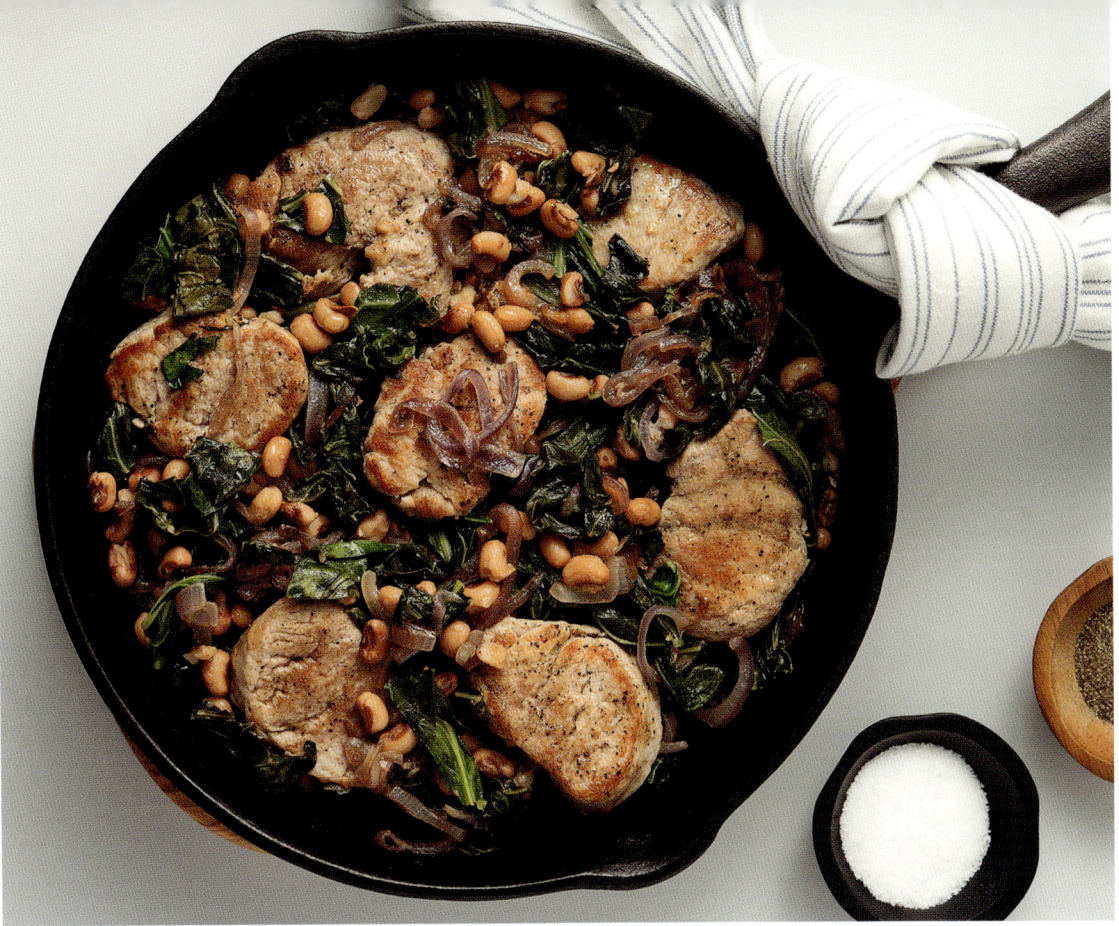

FOR THE PORK MEDALLIONS

1 pound (455 g) pork tenderloin

¼ teaspoon salt

¼ teaspoon ground black pepper

¼ teaspoon garlic powder

¼ teaspoon onion powder

1 tablespoon (15 ml) olive oil

TO MAKE THE PORK MEDALLIONS

While greens are cooking, slice pork into 8 roughly 2-ounce (55 g) pieces that resemble medallions. One at a time, place medallions into a plastic bag and flatten using a heavy object (like a hammer, rolling pin, or canned good) until the medallions are ¼ to ½-inch (0.6 to 1 cm) thick.

Combine salt, pepper, garlic powder, and onion powder together in a small bowl and sprinkle evenly over both sides of the pork medallions.

Heat olive oil in a large skillet over medium heat. Cook pork for 3 to 4 minutes on each side until it reaches an internal temperature of 145°F (63°C). This may require multiple batches depending on your pan size.

To serve, place one-quarter of greens in the center of each plate with 2 pork medallions on top.

CHILI

A common question that I receive is how to make a filling meal out of beans. My answer: Make a chili. The beautiful thing about chili is that it is always in season. Other soups and stews may lose favor in the warmer months, but chili always sounds good. And, of course, it's packed with beans! Since chili is naturally very low in fat, I added hemp seeds to my recipe to boost the healthy fats and provide additional protein.

■ **YIELD:**
4 SERVINGS

■ **PREP TIME:**
5 MINUTES

■ **COOK TIME:**
25 MINUTES

1 tablespoon (15 ml) olive oil

2 bell peppers, any color, diced

1 large onion, diced

1½ tablespoons (11.5 g) chili powder

1 teaspoon ground cumin

½ teaspoon ground coriander

½ teaspoon garlic powder

1 teaspoon salt

¼ teaspoon ground black pepper

2 garlic cloves, minced

2 (14.5-ounce [410 g]) cans diced tomatoes

2 tablespoons (32 g) tomato paste

1 cup (235 ml) chicken, beef, or vegetable broth

1 (15.5-ounce [423 g]) can pinto beans

1 (15.5-ounce [423 g]) can kidney beans

1 cup (130 g) frozen corn

½ cup (60 g) hemp seeds

OPTIONAL TOPPINGS

1 tablespoon (8 g) shredded cheddar cheese

Fresh cilantro

Diced red onion

Jalapeno slices

Avocado

Add olive oil, peppers, onions, chili powder, cumin, coriander, garlic powder, salt, and pepper to a large pot and sauté over medium-high heat for 10 minutes or until very soft. Add minced garlic and cook for 2 minutes before adding in tomatoes, tomato paste, broth, and beans. Bring to a simmer and allow to cook for 15 minutes. Stir in corn and hemp seeds.

Serve in a bowl with desired toppings.

NOTES

- Any canned beans work for this recipe. Feel free to substitute what you have.

- If adding shredded cheddar, 1 tablespoon (8 g) adds an additional 1.5 grams of saturated fat.

- Want to increase the protein? Add ½ pound (225 g) ground chicken or turkey after sautéing the vegetables to boost the protein content by 14 grams per serving.

NUTRITIONAL ANALYSIS

SERVING SIZE: About 2 cups (about 400 g) chili

PER SERVING: 440 calories; 14 g fat; 2 g saturated fat; 23 g protein; 610 g carbohydrates; 18 g dietary fiber

MINI MEATLOAVES WITH MASHED SWEET POTATOES AND GREEN BEANS

■ **YIELD:**
4 SERVINGS

■ **PREP TIME:**
10 MINUTES

■ **COOK TIME:**
20 MINUTES

Enjoy meatloaf without the hour or more of cooking time. When made in muffin form, meatloaf cooks much more quickly and can be on the dinner table in just 30 minutes.

Nonstick cooking spray

2 large sweet potatoes, peeled and cubed

½ teaspoon ground cinnamon

1 pound (455 g) ground chicken or turkey

¼ cup (28 g) ground flaxseed

1 tablespoon (15 ml) olive oil

1 teaspoon garlic powder

1 teaspoon onion powder

1 teaspoon salt, plus more as needed

¼ teaspoon ground black pepper

¼ cup (60 g) BBQ sauce

1 pound (455 g) fresh green beans, trimmed

Preheat oven to 375°F (190°C or gas mark 5) and place the rack in the center of the oven. Line a muffin pan with 8 standard muffin liners or silicon muffin cups. Spray each with nonstick spray.

Add sweet potatoes to a large pot of water. Bring to a boil over high heat and cook for 12 to 15 minutes or until you can easily press a fork into the potato, indicating they are soft enough to mash. Drain sweet potatoes and add them back to the hot pot. Mash with a potato masher and stir in cinnamon. Cover with a lid until the meatloaves have finished cooking.

While the sweet potatoes are cooking, make the meatloaves. Mix ground chicken or turkey with ground flaxseed, olive oil, garlic powder, onion powder, salt, and pepper in a large bowl until thoroughly combined. Evenly divide the mixture between the 8 lined muffin tins. Brush the tops with BBQ sauce. Cook in the oven for 18 to 20 minutes or until the internal cooking temperature reaches 165°F (74°C).

When the mini meatloaves have about 10 minutes left to cook, spray a skillet with nonstick spray and add green beans. Sauté on medium heat for 8 to 10 minutes until tender. Sprinkle with a dash of salt, if desired.

To serve, plate one-quarter of the sweet potato mash, 2 mini meatloaves, and one-quarter of the green beans. Enjoy!

NUTRITIONAL ANALYSIS

SERVING SIZE: 1 cup (240 g) mash + 2 meatloaves + ½ cup (about 112 g) green beans

PER SERVING: 554 calories; 28 g fat; 6 g saturated fat; 35 g protein; 44 g carbohydrates; 10 g dietary fiber

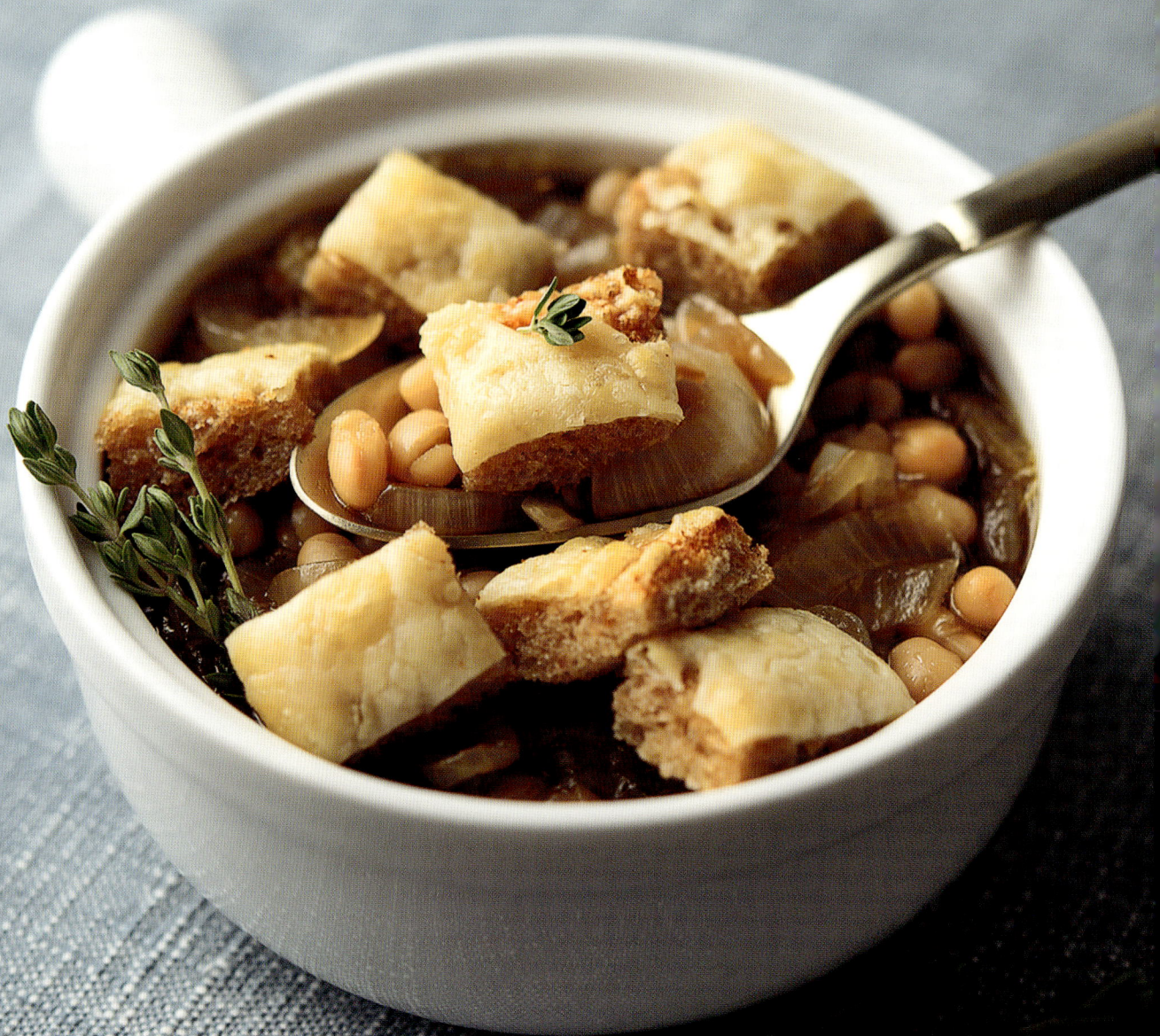

FRENCH ONION SOUP

Tuck into a warm, comforting bowl of French onion soup, a classic dish that features everything you need to satisfy your tastebuds and improve your cholesterol. It's got vegetables, beans to boost the fiber content, and cheesy croutons floating on top for a complete and filling meal.

■ YIELD:
4 SERVINGS

■ PREP TIME:
5 MINUTES

■ COOK TIME:
25 MINUTES

2 tablespoons (28 ml) olive oil

3 large onions, thinly sliced

1 teaspoon salt

¼ teaspoon ground black pepper

1 teaspoon dried thyme

8 ounces (225 g) baby portobella mushrooms, thinly sliced

4 cups (950 ml) low-sodium beef bone broth

2 (15.5-ounce [423 g]) cans navy beans, drained and rinsed

Worcestershire sauce to taste

¼ cup (25 g) grated Parmesan cheese, divided

¼ cup (30 g) grated Gruyère cheese, divided

4 slices whole wheat bread or baguette, thinly sliced

In a large stockpot, heat olive oil over medium-low heat. Add onions, salt, pepper, and thyme, and cook, stirring frequently, until onions are browned and very tender. After 10 minutes, add mushrooms. Continue cooking and stirring until the mushrooms are tender and brown and the onions are a dark brown, about 10 more minutes. Add beef broth and increase the heat to medium-high. Bring the soup to a simmer and add beans. Before serving, add 2 to 3 shakes (about 1 teaspoon [5 ml]) of Worcestershire sauce at a time, stir, and taste. The saltiness of your broth will influence how much is needed.

Arrange 1 tablespoon (5 g) Parmesan and 1 tablespoon (8 g) Gruyère on each slice of bread and place in a toaster or under a broiler. Once melted, cut bread into bite-size pieces.

To serve, ladle soup in a bowl and top with cheese toast.

NOTES

- Using beef bone broth in this recipe increases the protein content of the soup.

- Worcestershire sauce is a unique condiment that is hard to replicate. It is technically a fermented food made with anchovies, vinegar, sugar, garlic, onions, and spices. It increases the savory flavor of dishes. If you don't have it, just omit from the recipe.

NUTRITIONAL ANALYSIS

SERVING SIZE: 1½ cups (about 500 g) soup + 1 slice toast

PER SERVING: 305 calories; 12 g fat; 5 g saturated fat; 26 g protein; 34 g carbohydrates; 13 g dietary fiber

CHICKEN AND DUMPLINGS

This recipe was inspired by a student who took my course on lowering cholesterol, Ethel. She was brainstorming a way to make heart-healthy chicken and dumplings, which inspired me to try it out in my own kitchen.

■ **YIELD:**
4 SERVINGS

■ **PREP TIME:**
5 MINUTES

■ **COOK TIME:**
25 MINUTES

FOR THE STEW

3 celery stalks, diced

2 carrots, peeled and diced

1 large onion, diced

12 ounces (340 g) white mushrooms, sliced

1 tablespoon (15 ml) olive oil

1 teaspoon salt

1 teaspoon garlic powder

½ teaspoon ground black pepper

1 teaspoon dried thyme

1 teaspoon dried rosemary

3 cups (705 ml) chicken broth

½ cup (120 ml) cold water

¼ cup (31 g) flour

2 cups (280 g) cooked shredded chicken breasts

1 cup (130 g) frozen green peas

FOR THE DUMPLINGS

¾ cup (80 g) high-protein pancake mix or self-rising flour

½ teaspoon salt

½ teaspoon dried thyme

1 egg, beaten

¼ cup (60 ml) milk, divided

TO MAKE THE STEW

Add celery, carrots, onions, mushrooms, olive oil, salt, garlic powder, black pepper, thyme, rosemary, and chicken broth to the electric pressure cooker. Cook under high pressure for 8 minutes. Manually release pressure when time expires.

While the veggies are cooking in the electric pressure cooker, make a slurry by combining cold water and flour in a small bowl. Mix until the flour dissolves. Set aside.

TO MAKE THE DUMPLINGS

Next, prepare the dumpling mixture. Add pancake mix or self-rising flour, salt, and thyme to a bowl and mix to combine. Add egg and 2 tablespoons (28 ml) milk, and stir to thoroughly combine. Slowly add remaining 2 tablespoons (28 ml) milk, stirring, until you reach a waffle batter consistency that is relatively thick and scoopable. Set aside.

When the veggies are cooked, switch the electric pressure cooker to the sauté function. Add shredded chicken and peas and stir. Then add slurry mixture and stir to combine.

Gently place 8 evenly divided scoops of the dumpling mixture on top of the chicken stew. Cook the dumplings on one side for 3 minutes, then gently flip and cook them for another 3 minutes on the other side. Remove dumplings from the soup and divide them between 4 serving bowls. Spoon the chicken stew over the top, serve, and enjoy!

NUTRITIONAL ANALYSIS

SERVING SIZE: 2 dumplings + 1½ cups stew (about 400 g)

PER SERVING: 400 calories; 11 g fat; 2 g saturated fat; 35 g protein; 28 g carbohydrates; 5 g dietary fiber

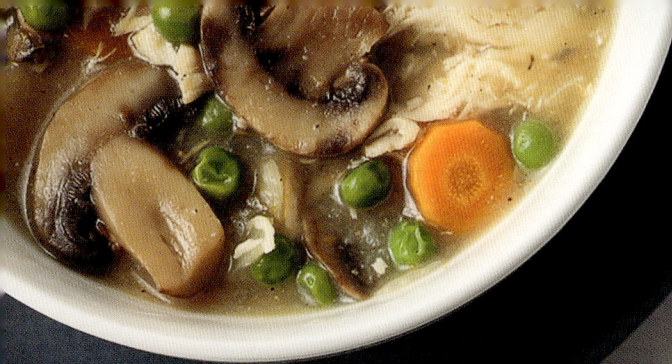

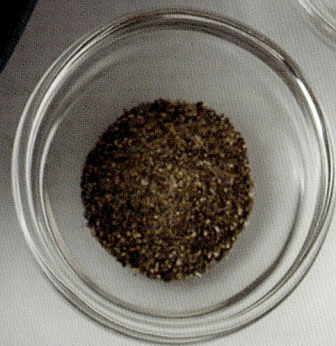

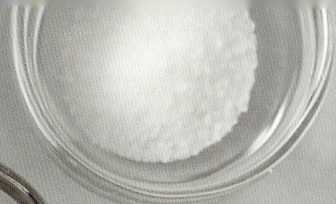

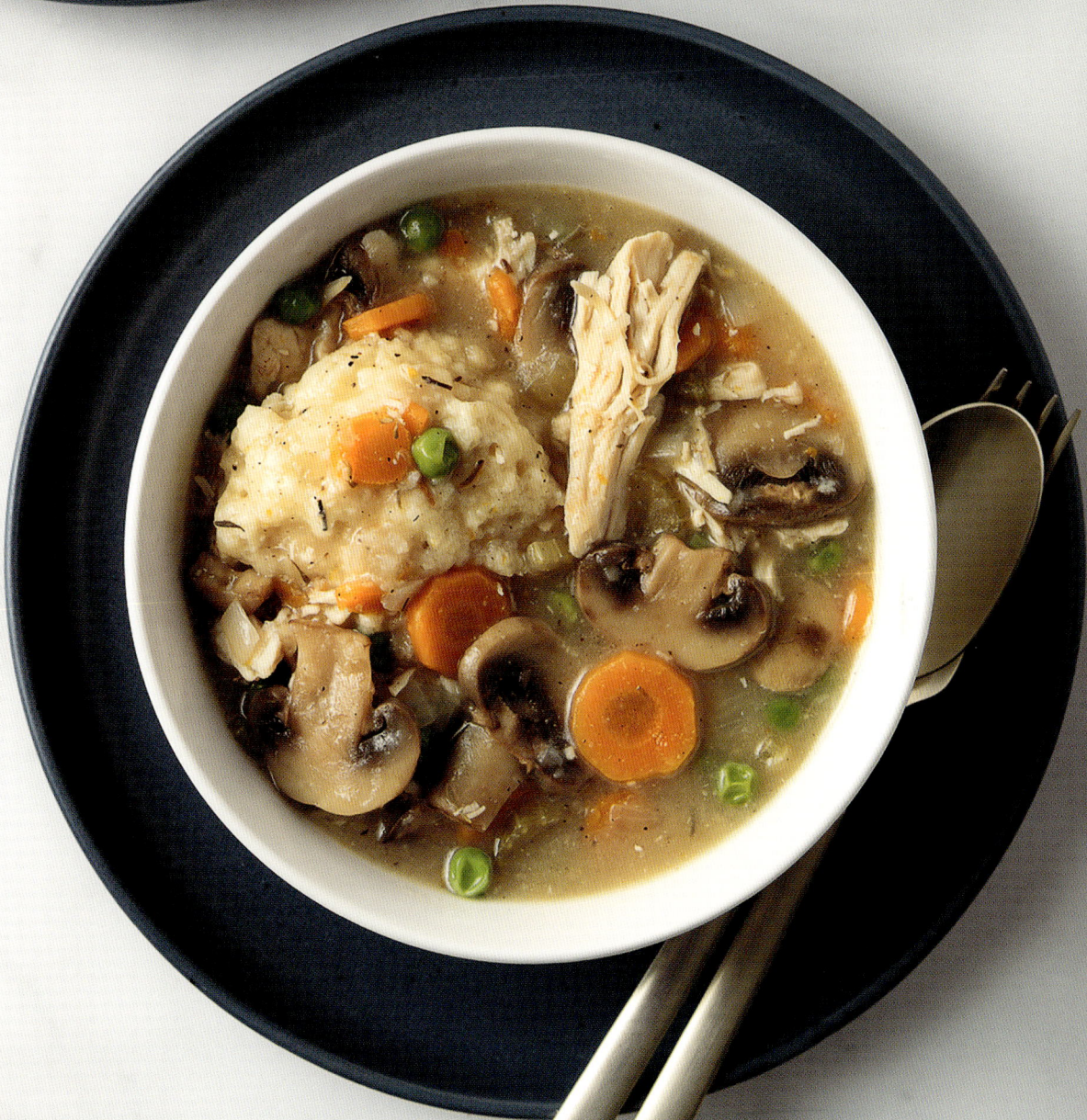

HARVEST CHICKEN SALAD

Cold, crisp greens and warm toppings make this salad the perfect candidate for a fall dinner. Featuring peppery arugula as the base, warming spices, sweet butternut squash, and tangy balsamic vinegar, this salad is both comforting and filling.

YIELD:
4 SERVINGS

PREP TIME:
5 MINUTES

COOK TIME:
25 MINUTES

- 1 pound (455 g) boneless, skinless chicken thighs, cut into 1-inch (2.5 cm) thick strips
- 1½ teaspoons olive oil
- ¼ teaspoon salt
- ¼ teaspoon ground black pepper
- ¼ teaspoon garlic
- 1 teaspoon dried thyme
- 2 cups (260 g) frozen butternut squash
- 1 small onion, thinly sliced
- 1 tablespoon (15 ml) olive oil
- ⅛ teaspoon ground cinnamon
- 1 (5-ounce [140 g]) container arugula
- ¼ cup (35 g) dried cranberries
- 1 (15.5-ounce [423 g]) can navy beans, drained and rinsed
- ¼ cup (16 g) pumpkin seeds
- 1 tablespoon (15 ml) balsamic vinegar or glaze

Preheat oven to 400°F (200°C or gas mark 6) and place a rack in the center. Arrange chicken on one side of a large baking sheet lined with parchment paper or a silicon baking sheet. Coat with olive oil and seasonings. On the other side of the baking sheet, arrange squash and onions. Mix with olive oil and cinnamon.

Bake for 22 minutes or until the chicken thighs reach an internal temperature of 165°F (74°C).

Arrange arugula at the bottom of a large dish. Add cranberries, beans, and pumpkin seeds. When chicken is finished, slide entire contents of baking sheet on top of the arugula. Drizzle with balsamic vinegar or glaze. Gently toss and serve.

NUTRITIONAL ANALYSIS

SERVING SIZE: About 2¼ cups (about 300 g) salad

PER SERVING: 436 calories; 21 g fat; 5 g saturated fat; 29 g protein; 35 g carbohydrates; 8 g dietary fiber

NOTE

Yes, you can roast vegetables from frozen! Preheat the oven to 400°F (200°C or gas mark 6) and check them after 20 minutes.

PUMPKIN LENTIL SOUP

■ YIELD:
2 SERVINGS

■ PREP TIME:
5 MINUTES

■ COOK TIME:
25 MINUTES

Quick-cooking red lentils bring this soup together in under 30 minutes. Lentils are an excellent source of protein and fiber that essentially dissolve in the soup, creating a creamy and filling texture. The pumpkin in this recipe provides over 100 percent of your daily recommended amount of vitamin A in the form of beta-carotene, a potent antioxidant that can help to manage inflammation. Paired with dried spices and cilantro, it is a delight for your tastebuds and cholesterol markers.

- 1 tablespoon (15 ml) olive oil
- ½ red onion, diced
- ½ teaspoon salt
- ½ teaspoon ground cumin
- ½ teaspoon ground turmeric
- ¼ teaspoon ground smoked paprika
- ¼ teaspoon ground ginger
- ¼ teaspoon ground black pepper
- 2 garlic cloves, minced
- 4 cups (950 ml) low-sodium chicken broth
- 1 cup (245 g) pureed pumpkin
- 1 cup (192 g) red lentils
- ¼ cup (4 g) fresh cilantro

Add olive oil to a medium saucepan and heat over medium-high heat. Add onion, salt, cumin, turmeric, paprika, ginger, and black pepper. Sauté for 8 to 10 minutes until onions are tender. Add in garlic and sauté for 2 more minutes, then add broth, pumpkin, and lentils. Bring to a boil and reduce to a simmer for 15 to 20 minutes or until lentils are completely soft, stirring occasionally. Serve in a bowl garnished with fresh cilantro.

NUTRITIONAL ANALYSIS

SERVING SIZE: 2 cups (about 450 g) soup

PER SERVING: 346 calories; 6 g fat; 1 g saturated fat; 18 g protein; 51 g carbohydrates; 21 g dietary fiber

NOTE

If you prefer a thicker soup, reduce the broth to 3½ cups (784 ml).

CRISPY TOFU WITH COCONUT RICE AND MANGO SLAW

■ **YIELD:**
4 SERVINGS

■ **PREP TIME:**
5 MINUTES

■ **COOK TIME:**
25 MINUTES

If you are skeptical about tofu, making it crispy in the oven is a great way to try it first. When tossed with a small amount of cornstarch, the texture of the tofu completely changes. The seasonings in this recipe really make it a pleasant explosion of flavor too. Paired with a light mango slaw and coconut rice, this meal is balanced and a delicious way to lower your cholesterol.

FOR THE TOFU

- 1 (15-ounce [420 g]) block high-protein, extra-firm tofu (see Notes)
- 1 tablespoon (15 ml) avocado oil
- 2 tablespoons (28 ml) soy sauce
- 1 tablespoon (8 g) cornstarch
- ¼ teaspoon ground black pepper
- ½ teaspoon garlic powder
- ½ teaspoon onion powder
- ¼ teaspoon ground ginger

FOR THE COCONUT RICE

- 1 cup (158 g) white rice, rinsed
- 2 cups (475 ml) boxed coconut milk or coconut almond milk (see Notes)

TO MAKE THE TOFU

Preheat oven to 425°F (220°C or gas mark 7). Place rack in the middle of the oven.

Slice tofu into 1-inch (2.5 cm) long, ½-inch (1 cm) thick rectangles. Pat the tofu dry with a paper towel. In a medium bowl, mix tofu with avocado oil, soy sauce, cornstarch, and seasonings. Spread pieces evenly onto a baking sheet with the long, flat side of the tofu facing down. Bake on the middle rack for 25 minutes, turning after 15 minutes.

TO MAKE THE RICE

In a medium saucepan, bring rice and coconut milk to a boil. Reduce to a simmer and cover for 8 to 10 minutes until liquid is absorbed and rice is light and fluffy.

NOTES

- Tofu comes in a range of firmness: silken or soft, medium, firm, extra-firm, and high-protein. The difference between these is simply how much water has been expelled from the block of tofu. This recipe works best with high-protein tofu, which is the firmest type. If you cannot find high-protein, then pressing your tofu will help to expel extra water. Wrap it in a towel and place under something heavy for 30 minutes.

- Making the rice with boxed or almond-coconut milk instead of canned coconut milk drastically reduces the saturated fat typically found in coconut rice. Using this method, you can still enjoy the coconut flavor without the coconut fat.

NUTRITIONAL ANALYSIS

SERVING SIZE: ½ cup (79 g) rice + ¾ cup (about 130 g) slaw + ¾ cup (about 105 g) tofu

PER SERVING: 507 calories; 19 g fat; 5 g saturated fat; 24 g protein; 61 g carbohydrates; 7 g dietary fiber

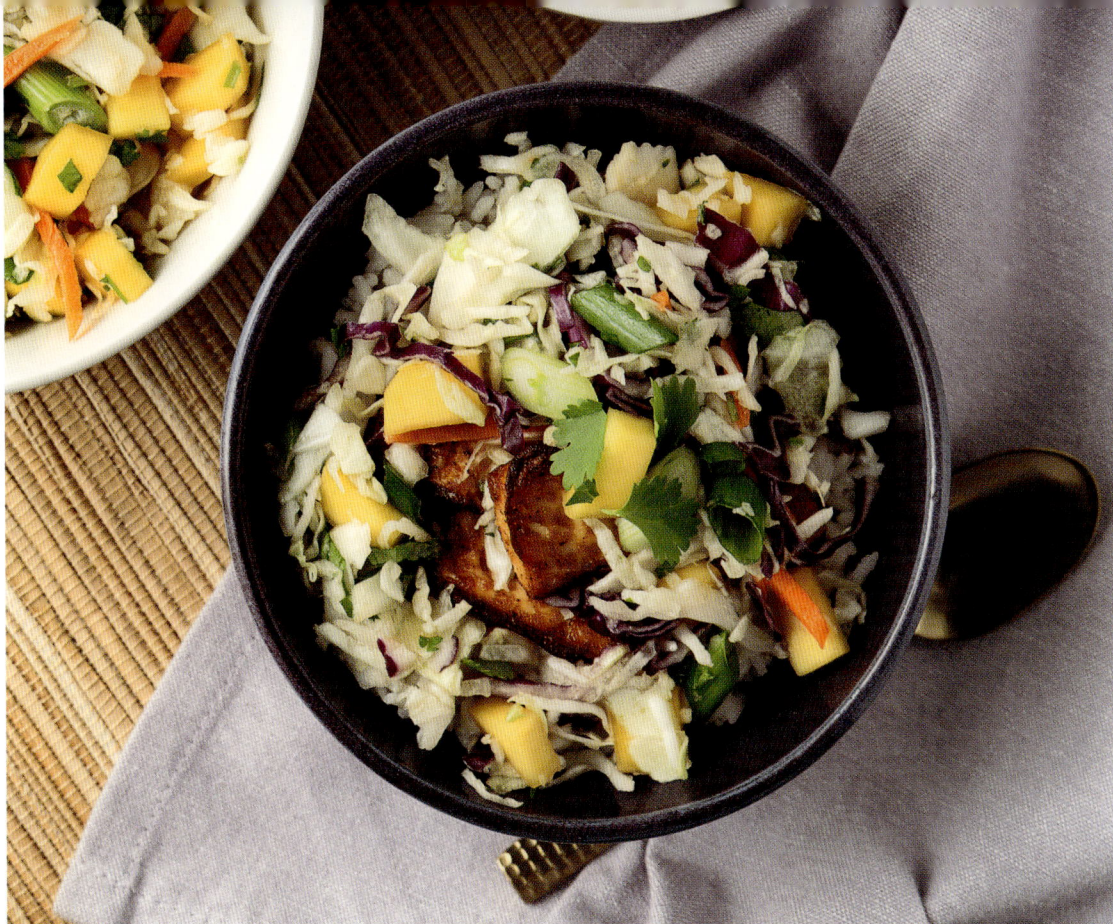

FOR THE MANGO SLAW

1 cup (175 g) fresh or frozen
mango

1½ teaspoons avocado oil

1½ teaspoons sesame oil

2 teaspoons fish sauce

12 ounces (340 g) cabbage or
broccoli slaw

4 green onions, both green and
white parts, minced

¼ cup (4 g) fresh cilantro

½ teaspoon sugar or honey
(depends on sweetness of
mango), if needed

TO MAKE THE MANGO SLAW

While the rice and tofu are cooking, make the slaw. Cut mango into small, bite-size pieces. Place at the bottom of a large bowl. Add oils and fish sauce and toss to combine. Then add slaw, green onions, and cilantro. Toss until everything is thoroughly coated. The slaw should taste slightly sweet and balanced (not too salty) because of the mango. If it is not, add sugar or honey and toss to combine.

To serve, plate one-quarter of the rice in the bottom of a bowl. Then add one-quarter of the tofu and top with one-quarter of the slaw. Enjoy!

SEITAN "BEEF" AND BROCCOLI

Try your hand at takeout at home. Seitan has a texture similar to meat and can fool most meat eaters when covered in this delicious sauce. If you can't find seitan, you can freeze a block of tofu, thaw it, and slice it into thin rectangles to achieve a similar texture.

YIELD:
3 SERVINGS

PREP TIME:
5 MINUTES

COOK TIME:
20 MINUTES

¾ cup (119 g) white rice

1½ tablespoons (25 ml) avocado oil

2 cups (312 g) frozen broccoli

1 (8-ounce [227 g]) package seitan, sliced

3 green onions, both green and white parts, sliced

2 garlic cloves, grated

½-inch (1 cm) piece fresh ginger, grated

1½ tablespoons (25 ml) soy sauce

1 tablespoon (15 g) brown sugar

2 tablespoons (28 ml) water

2 teaspoons cornstarch

Prepare rice according to package instructions.

While rice is cooking, add avocado oil to a large skillet. Heat over medium-high heat and add frozen broccoli. Cook for 2 to 3 minutes before moving it to the side of the pan. Add seitan and sear on both sides for 2 to 3 minutes or until a slight crisp forms. Stir broccoli occasionally to ensure it doesn't burn.

Add green onions, garlic, and ginger to the pan. Cook for 2 minutes until it becomes fragrant, then add soy sauce and brown sugar. Make a cornstarch slurry by mixing together the water and cornstarch in a small bowl or jar. Add the slurry to the pan and bring to a boil for 2 minutes to thicken the sauce.

Serve the "beef" and broccoli over rice.

NOTES

- Not sure about seitan? It is one of the original plant-based proteins. It is made from wheat gluten, the same type of protein found in wheat baked goods. Seitan is made from essentially washing away the starch of bread dough until only the high-protein gluten remains. It is very versatile because it has no flavor, has a dense and meaty texture, and is shelf stable. It makes a great meat substitute in strongly flavored dishes like this one.

- Add 1½ cups (255 g) frozen shelled edamame while cooking to add 11 grams of protein and 9 grams of fiber.

NUTRITIONAL ANALYSIS

SERVING SIZE: ½ cup (83 g) rice + 1 cup (about 130 g) seitan and broccoli

PER SERVING: 422 calories; 8 g fat; 1 g saturated fat; 21 g protein; 45 g carbohydrates; 4 g dietary fiber

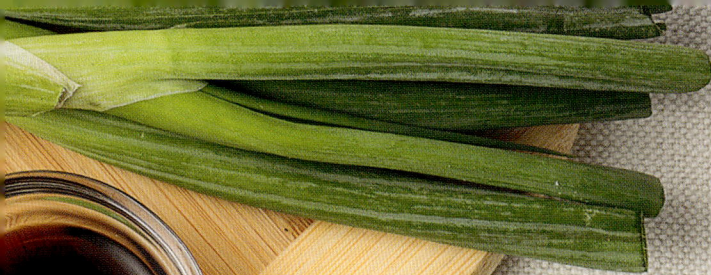

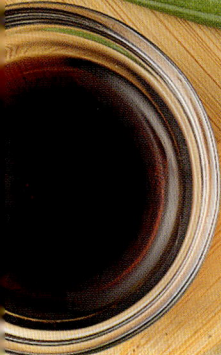

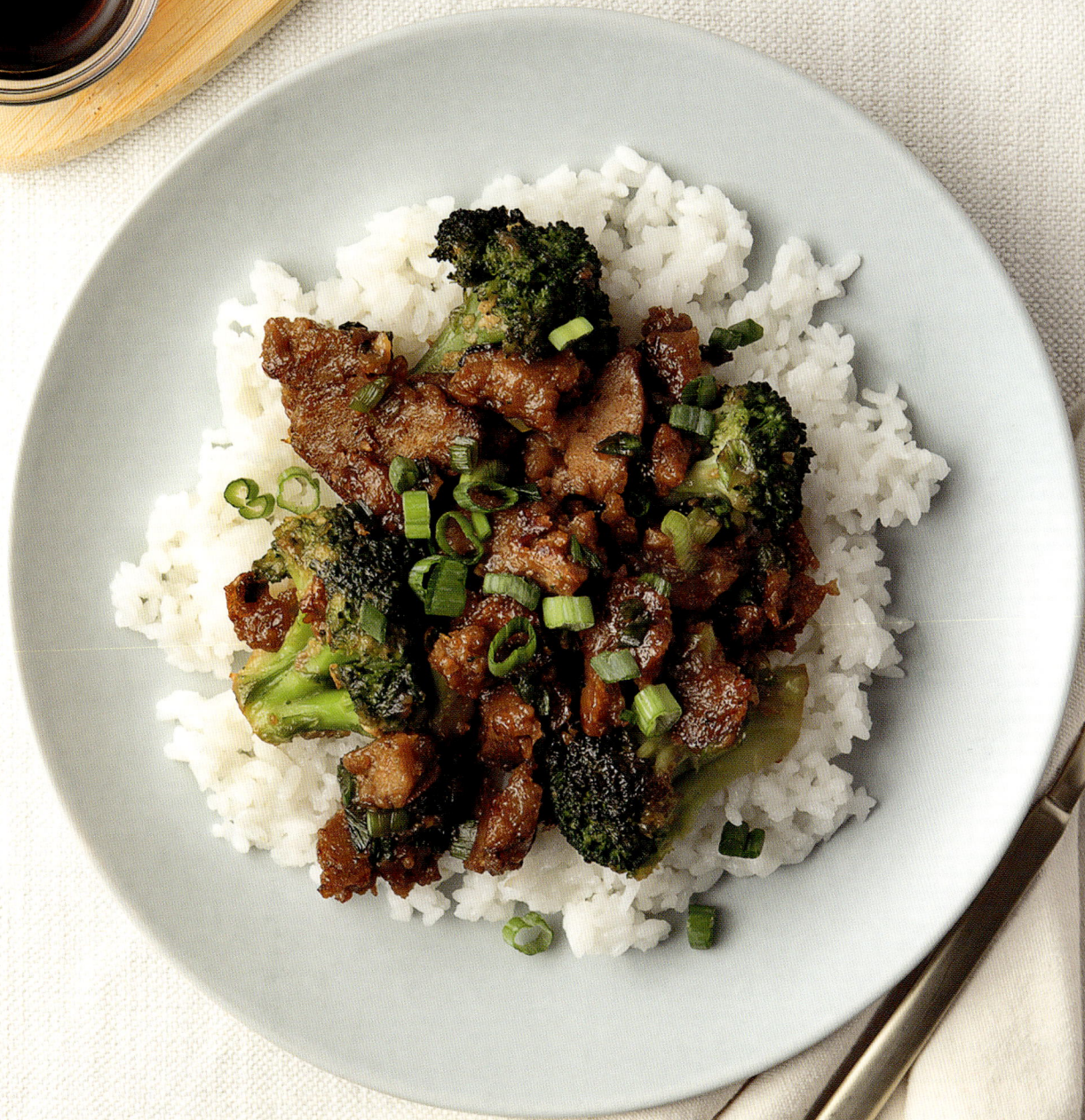

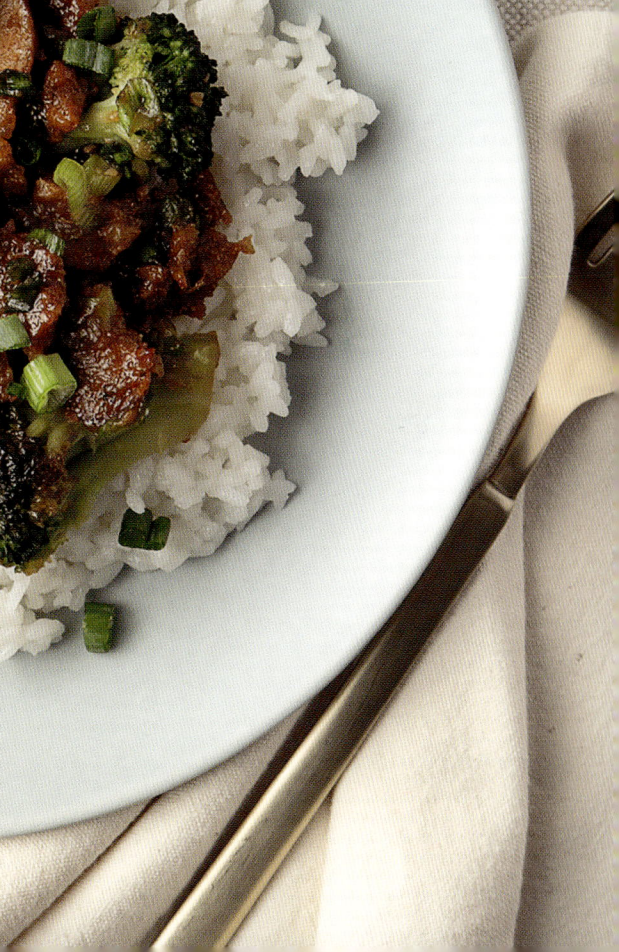

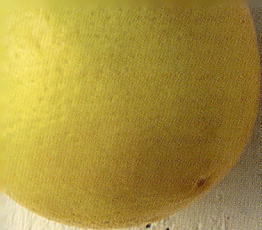

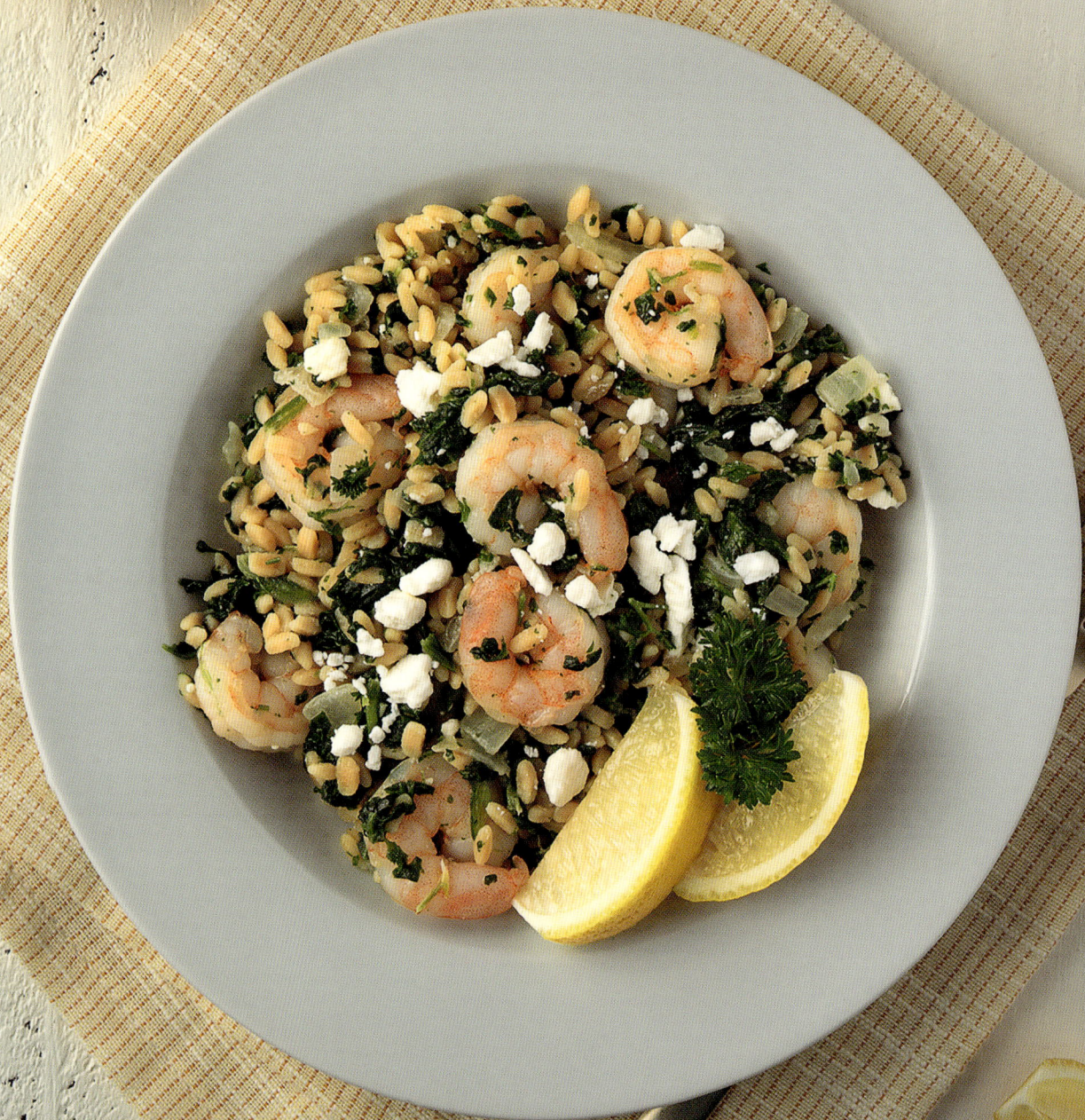

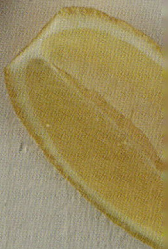

SPANAKOPITA SHRIMP BOWLS

A fun twist on the Greek dish spanakopita that highlights spinach, feta, and parsley, this recipe uses high-fiber rice and lean-protein shrimp to make a complete, cholesterol-friendly meal.

■ **YIELD:**
4 SERVINGS

■ **PREP TIME:**
5 MINUTES

■ **COOK TIME:**
25 MINUTES

1 (8-ounce [225 g]) bag bean-based rice, like Banza

1 tablespoon (15 ml) olive oil

1 medium onion, diced

1 pound (455 g) shrimp, peeled and deveined

2 cups (360 g) frozen spinach

3 garlic cloves, minced

¼ cup (60 ml) chicken broth

½ cup (30 g) fresh parsley

¼ cup (38 g) feta cheese

1 teaspoon lemon juice

Salt, to taste

Prepare bean-based rice according to package instructions. Once cooked, rinse and set aside.

Heat olive oil in a medium skillet or sauté pan over medium-high heat. Add onion and sauté for 7 to 8 minutes or until tender. Add shrimp and sauté for 1 minute on each side before adding spinach and garlic. Continue cooking until spinach is completely thawed and heated through, about 5 minutes. Add chicken broth and bring to a low simmer.

Turn off heat and stir in parsley, feta cheese, lemon juice, and rice. Add to a shallow bowl and enjoy!

NUTRITIONAL ANALYSIS

SERVING SIZE: About 1 cup (about 250 g) rice, spinach, and shrimp mixture

PER SERVING: 538 calories; 17 g fat; 3 g saturated fat; 37 g protein; 64 g carbohydrates; 13 g dietary fiber

AIR-FRYER SALMON BITES WITH CAULIFLOWER STIR-FRY

■ YIELD:
4 SERVINGS

■ PREP TIME:
15 MINUTES

■ COOK TIME:
15 MINUTES

These crispy salmon bites are not only delicious but also provide you with a healthy dose of heart-healthy omega-3 fats. Paired with an easy stir-fry, this meal will be on your dinner table often!

FOR THE SALMON

1 pound (455 g) fresh salmon, cut into 1-inch (2.5 cm) cubes

2 tablespoons (28 ml) soy sauce

2 tablespoons (40 g) maple syrup

2 tablespoons (28 ml) avocado oil

FOR THE STIR-FRY

1 teaspoon avocado oil

2 heads cauliflower, cut into florets

3 garlic cloves, minced

2 cups (316 g) cooked brown rice

¼ cup (60 ml) water

1 tablespoon (15 ml) soy sauce

1½ teaspoons sesame oil

2 green onions, both green and white parts, thinly sliced

Sesame seeds for garnish

TO MAKE THE SALMON

In a medium bowl, combine salmon with soy sauce, maple syrup, and avocado oil. Set aside to marinate for 15 minutes. When salmon has finished marinating, add it to the air fryer and cook on 400°F (200°C) for 8 minutes. If you don't have an air fryer, you can bake these in a 400°F (200°C or gas mark 6) oven, turning halfway through, for 8 to 10 minutes or until the center is opaque.

TO MAKE THE STIR-FRY

In the meantime, prepare the vegetables. Heat avocado oil in a large skillet. Add cauliflower and sauté over medium-high heat for 8 to 10 minutes, or until it begins to become tender. Add garlic and sauté for 2 additional minutes. Then add brown rice, water, and soy sauce. Sauté for 4 to 5 minutes or until rice is heated through. Remove from heat and garnish with sesame oil and green onions.

Plate your stir-fry and add salmon bites on top. Garnish with sesame seeds and serve.

NUTRITIONAL ANALYSIS

SERVING SIZE: 1 cup (about 80 g) salmon + 1 cup (about 200 g) stir-fry

PER SERVING: 473 calories; 18 g fat; 2 g saturated fat; 38 g protein; 40 g carbohydrates; 4 g dietary fiber

NOTE

The salmon bites also taste great cold the next day. Eat them wrapped in seaweed for a sushi-style lunch.

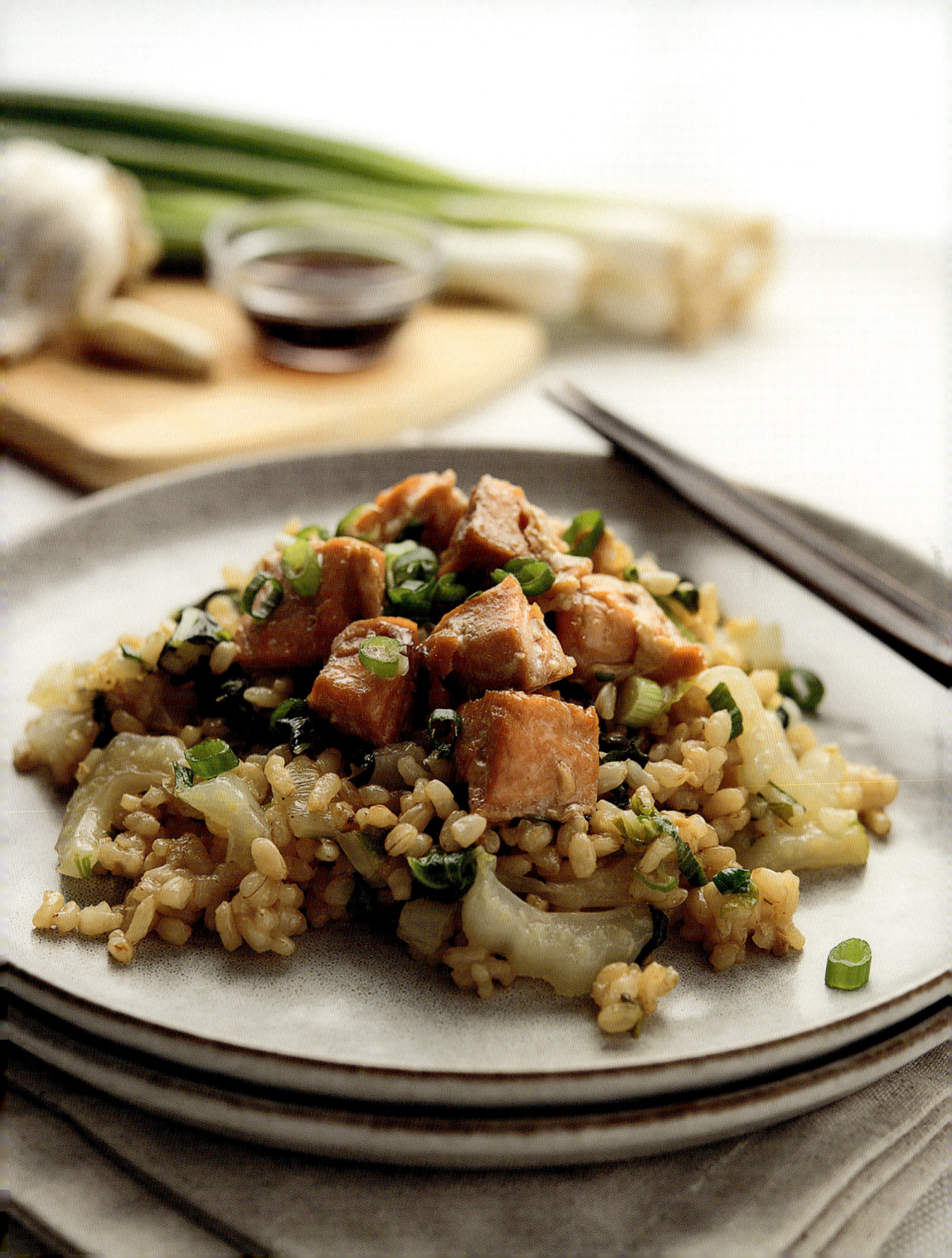

SHRIMP AND GRITS

■ **YIELD:**
4 SERVINGS

■ **PREP TIME:**
5 MINUTES

■ **COOK TIME:**
20 MINUTES

Most shrimp and grits recipes are incredibly tasty due to the incredible amount of butter they contain. Unfortunately, this is not ideal for cholesterol levels. In lieu of butter, this recipe uses olive oil, garlic, cherry tomatoes, and Cajun seasoning to make this classic dish heart-healthier while still maintaining a delicious taste. Shrimp is a fast-cooking and lean source of protein that is great to include in your diet, even though, like all animal proteins, it does include some dietary cholesterol.

- **1½ tablespoons (25 ml) olive oil**
- **2 bunches kale, chopped, about 8 cups (536 g)**
- **½ red onion, thinly sliced**
- **4 garlic cloves, minced**
- **1 cup (150 g) cherry tomatoes, halved**
- **1 pound (455 g) peeled and deveined frozen shrimp**
- **1 cup (140 g) quick-cooking polenta**
- **2 tablespoons (10 g) grated Parmesan cheese**
- **1½ teaspoons Cajun, creole, or seafood seasoning**

Add olive oil, kale, and red onion to a large sauté pan and cook over medium heat, stirring frequently, for 10 minutes, or until the kale is completely wilted and the onions are tender. Add garlic and cherry tomatoes. Sauté for 5 minutes, then remove from the pan and set aside. Add frozen shrimp to the pan. Cook for 4 minutes on each side or until the shrimp are opaque.

While the shrimp are cooking, cook polenta according to package instructions. When polenta has absorbed all of the water, remove from heat and stir in Parmesan cheese.

When shrimp are finished cooking, add the vegetable mixture back to the pan and add Cajun seasoning. Toss to evenly distribute the seasoning.

To serve, add one-quarter of the cooked polenta to the bottom of a bowl. Top with one-quarter of the shrimp mixture.

NUTRITIONAL ANALYSIS

SERVING SIZE: 1 cup (250 g) polenta + 1 cup (about 300 g) shrimp mixture

PER SERVING: 402 calories; 9 g fat; 1 g saturated fat; 35 g protein; 46 g carbohydrates; 5 g dietary fiber

NOTE

What's the difference between polenta and grits? Both are made from corn, but typically different varieties. Grits usually have a finer texture and result in a smoother porridge-like consistency. Polenta has a coarser, flakier texture. Polenta makes a nicer base for this recipe.

PORK TENDERLOIN WITH MUSHROOM GRAVY AND RICE

■ **YIELD:**
4 SERVINGS

■ **PREP TIME:**
10 MINUTES

■ **COOK TIME:**
20 MINUTES

Pork chops with mushroom gravy always reminds me of my childhood. It was a staple in our house and one of the first recipes I knew I wanted to add to this cookbook. Using pork tenderloin instead of pork chops reduces the saturated-fat content and drastically speeds up the cooking time. The gravy is also made from scratch instead of using cream of mushroom soup, further reducing the fat content.

1 cup (158 g) brown rice

1 pound (455 g) pork tenderloin, cut into 1-inch (2.5 cm) cubes

½ teaspoon salt

½ teaspoon ground black pepper

½ teaspoon garlic powder

2 tablespoons (30 ml) olive oil, divided

8–12 ounces (225–340 g) sliced mushrooms

1 large onion, thinly sliced

1 tablespoon (8 g) flour

1½ cups (355 ml) chicken stock

Worcestershire sauce, to taste

4 cups (624 g) fresh or frozen broccoli

Prepare brown rice according to package directions. Set aside.

While the rice is cooking, add pork tenderloin to a large bowl and toss with salt, pepper, and garlic powder. Set aside. In a large skillet, add 1 tablespoon (15 ml) olive oil, mushrooms, and onions. Cook over medium heat until onions and mushrooms are brown and tender, about 10 minutes. Then add in pork and cook for 3 to 4 minutes. Stir and cook for another 3 to 4 minutes.

Add the remaining tablespoon (15 ml) of olive oil to the skillet, then sprinkle in flour. Stir to combine and cook for 2 to 3 minutes, or until flour starts to bubble. Then slowly pour in chicken stock while stirring vigorously to prevent clumps. Continue stirring over medium heat until sauce begins to bubble and thicken, about 5 minutes. Then add Worcestershire sauce to taste. I use 1 to 2 shakes (about ½ teaspoon).

While the sauce is cooking, microwave broccoli for 3 minutes.

Plate the brown rice and broccoli. Spoon the pork tenderloin and sauce over the rice and serve.

NOTE

I mentioned in the introduction that not every recipe will be "perfect" when it comes to lowering your cholesterol. This one is on the lower side for dietary fiber, but it is a drastic improvement nutritionally from the original recipe. When building your daily menus, take note of high- versus low-fiber meals. This dish would be the perfect dinner after a high-fiber bean-based lunch, like the Three Bean Salad with Edamame (page 63).

NUTRITIONAL ANALYSIS

SERVING SIZE: ½ cup (79 g) rice + 1 cup (156 g) broccoli + ¾ cup (about 300 g) pork with sauce

PER SERVING: 462 calories; 13 g fat; 3 g saturated fat; 33 g protein; 51 g carbohydrates; 5 g dietary fiber

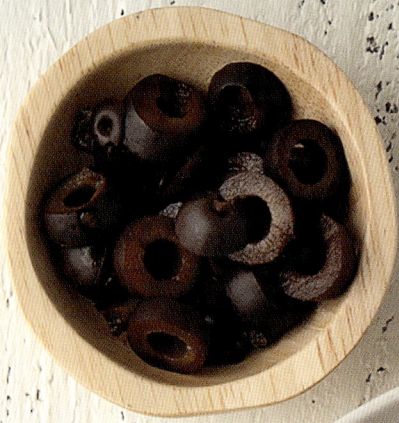

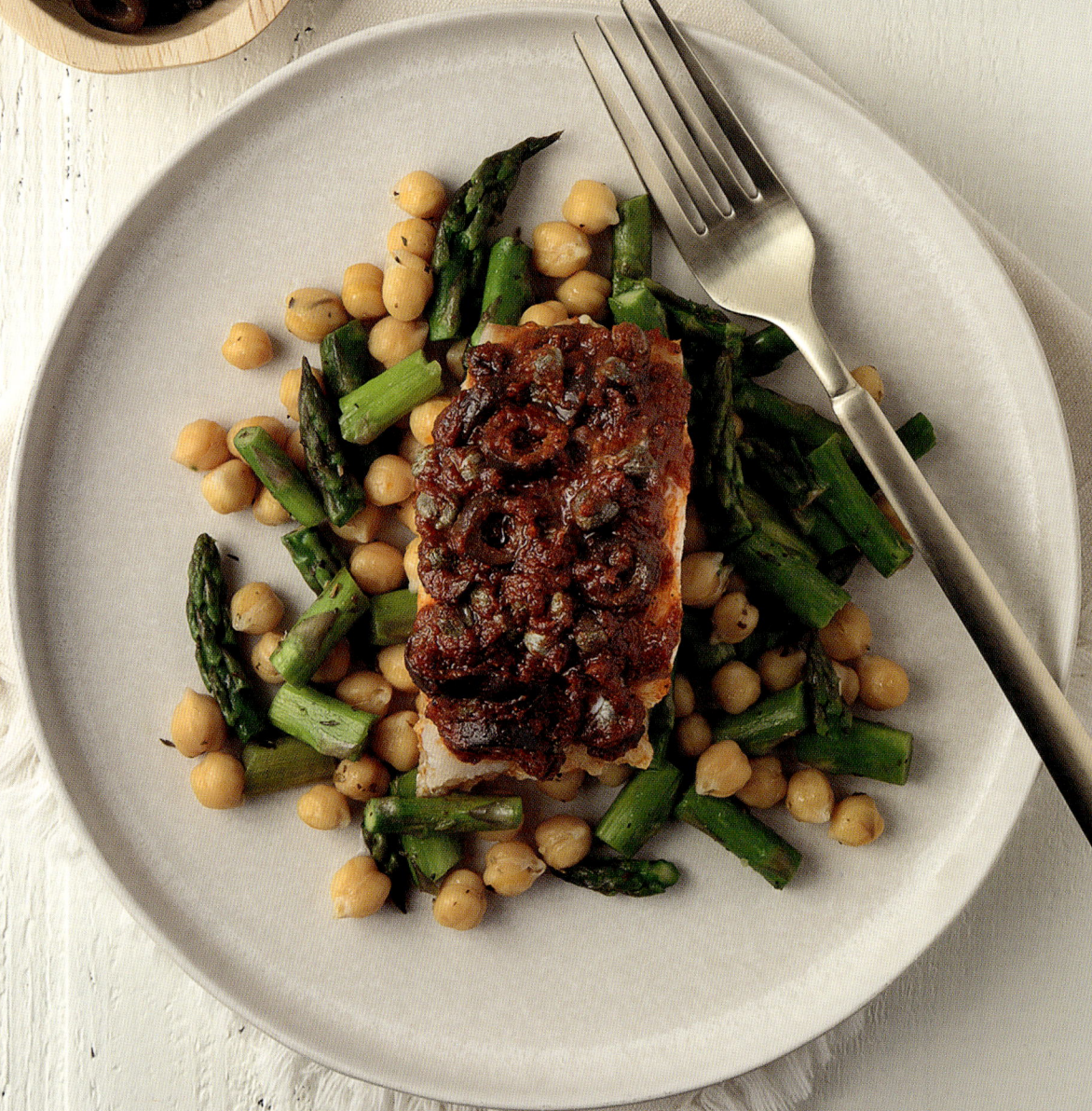

COD PUTTANESCA WITH ASPARAGUS AND CHICKPEAS

■ **YIELD:**
4 SERVINGS

■ **PREP TIME:**
5 MINUTES

■ **COOK TIME:**
20 MINUTES

The mild taste of cod is made more exciting by this flavorful puttanesca topping. Sweet tomato paste, salty olives and capers, and aromatic garlic powder combine to create a complex and mouthwatering sauce. Paired with high-fiber asparagus and chickpeas, this is a light but filling meal that is great for your heart. It also tastes great with bean-based pasta.

2 tablespoons (32 g) tomato paste

2 tablespoons (28 ml) olive oil

2 tablespoons (13 g) sliced black olives or olive tapenade

2 tablespoons (17 g) capers

½ teaspoon garlic powder

¼ teaspoon ground black pepper

1 pound (455 g) cod fillet

1½ teaspoons olive oil

1 pound (455 g) asparagus, chopped into 1-inch (2.5 cm) pieces

2 (15.5-ounce [423 g]) cans chickpeas, drained and rinsed

½ teaspoon salt

1 teaspoon Italian seasoning

Preheat oven to 375°F (190°C or gas mark 5) and place a rack in the center. Line a baking sheet with parchment paper or silicone mats.

In a small bowl, mix together tomato paste, olive oil, olives or tapenade, capers, garlic powder, and black pepper. Arrange cod on the prepared baking sheet and spread puttanesca sauce evenly on top of the fillet. Bake for 12 to 14 minutes or until the fish is opaque throughout and flakes easily.

While the fish is cooking, add olive oil to a large skillet. Sauté asparagus over medium heat until it becomes tender, about 5 minutes. Add chickpeas, salt, and Italian seasonings. Sauté for 5 additional minutes until chickpeas are heated through.

To serve, plate chickpeas and asparagus and place cod on top. Enjoy!

NUTRITIONAL ANALYSIS

SERVING SIZE: 1 4-ounce (114 g) cod fillet with sauce + 1 cup (about 200 g) chickpea mix

PER SERVING: 406 calories; 15 g fat; 2 g saturated fat; 36 g protein; 37 g carbohydrates; 13 g dietary fiber

WALNUT HONEY MUSTARD SALMON WITH BABY BROCCOLI

YIELD:
4 SERVINGS

PREP TIME:
10 MINUTES

COOK TIME:
20 MINUTES

Inspired by the popular dish at American Chinese restaurants, this dish packs the flavor of honey walnut shrimp without the deep-fried and sugar-heavy components of the meal. Getting in your omega-3s has never been so tasty.

- 2 cups (475) water
- 1 cup (184 g) quinoa, rinsed
- 3 tablespoons (60 g) honey
- 3 tablespoons (33 g) brown or Dijon mustard
- 1 tablespoon (15 ml) olive oil
- ½ cup (120 g) chopped walnuts
- Nonstick spray
- 1 pound (455 g) salmon (4 fillets)
- ⅛ teaspoon salt
- 1 pound (455 g) baby broccoli or broccolini, or frozen broccoli (see Note)

Preheat oven to 375°F (190°C or gas mark 5) and place rack in the center.

Bring water to a boil in a medium saucepan. Once boiling, add quinoa and reduce to a simmer. Cover and allow to simmer until all water has been absorbed, about 15 minutes.

In a small bowl, mix together honey, mustard, olive oil, and walnuts. Spray a baking sheet with nonstick cooking spray. Arrange salmon on one-half of the baking sheet. Sprinkle with salt, then evenly spread honey walnut mixture over salmon. On the other side of the sheet, lay out baby broccoli in an even layer. Bake for 14 to 16 minutes or until salmon is an opaque pink color throughout.

Spread quinoa evenly over your plate. Place broccoli in the center and then place salmon on top.

NOTE

While very similar to broccoli, baby broccoli is actually a different plant. It also goes by the name broccolini or tender-stem broccoli and typically has smaller florets and much longer stems than broccoli. It is ideal for a quick-cooking recipe as it gets tender very quickly when roasted. If you can't find baby broccoli or broccolini, substitute frozen broccoli. Frozen vegetables are preblanched, which helps them to cook more quickly.

NUTRITIONAL ANALYSIS

SERVING SIZE: ¾ cup (150 g) quinoa + 1 cup (71 g) broccoli + 1 salmon fillet

PER SERVING: 458 calories; 24 g fat; 4 g saturated fat; 32 g protein; 31 g carbohydrates; 8 g dietary fiber

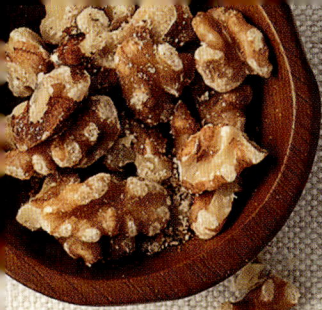

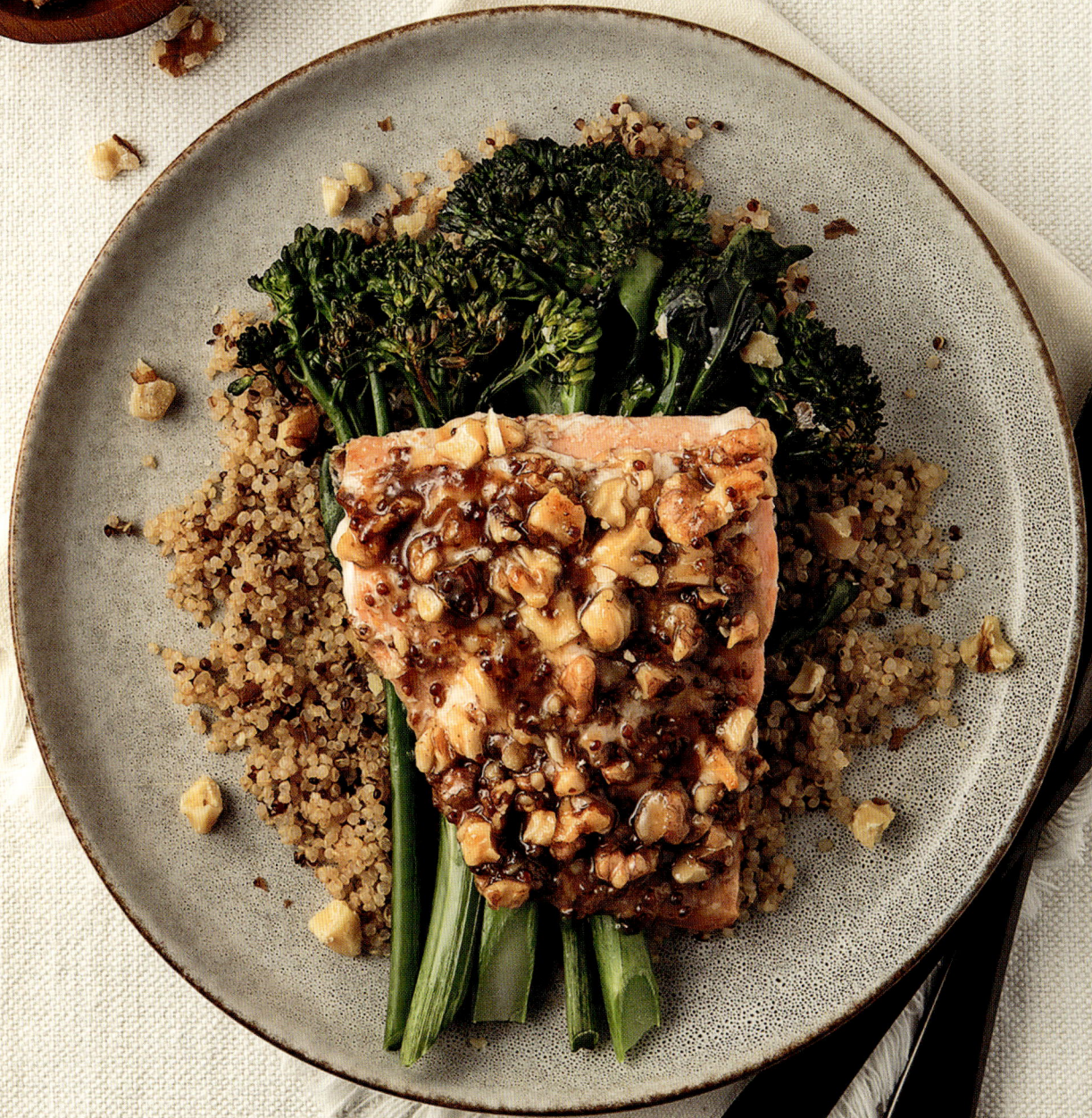

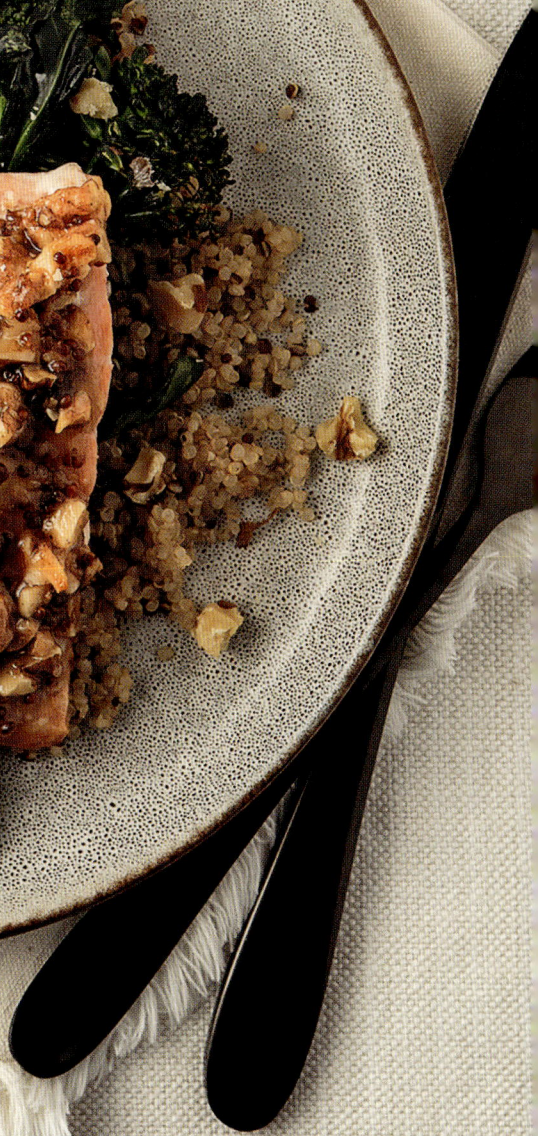

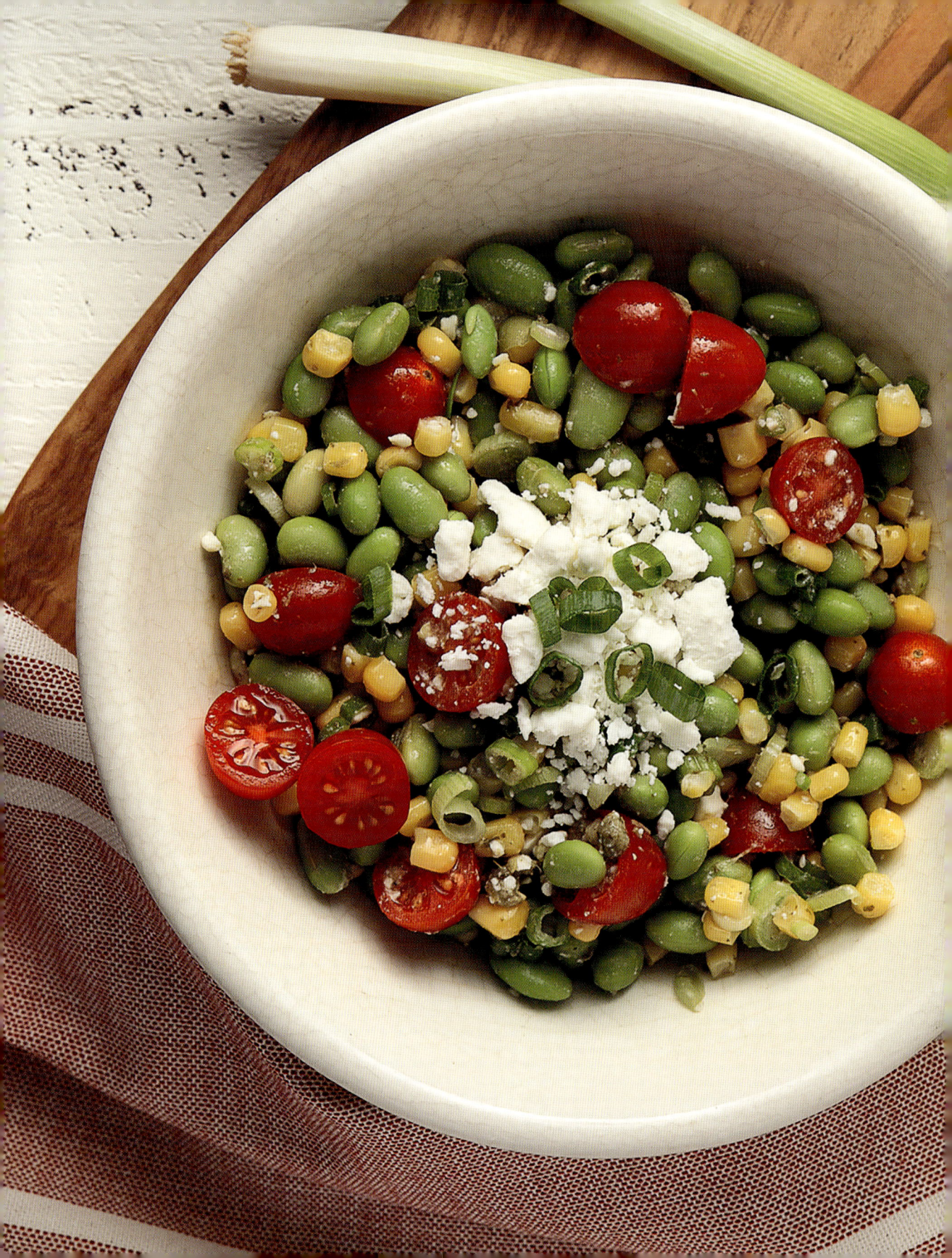

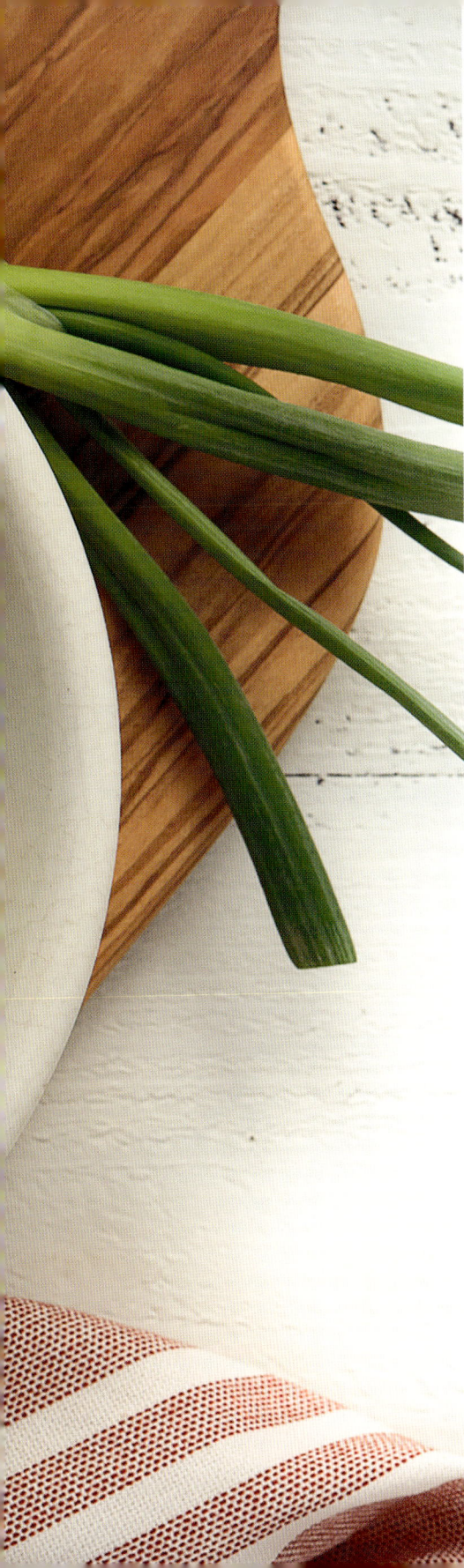

CHAPTER 6

10 Snacks and Treats in 10 Minutes

Snacks and treats are a part of any balanced diet and can definitely play a role in helping you meet your nutrient goals and lower your cholesterol. The options in this chapter all serve a purpose—whether that is to boost your fiber intake, help you eat enough protein, satisfy a sweet tooth responsibly, or help you get in some much-needed nutrients on "off" days. These recipes were developed to keep your cravings satisfied and your cholesterol levels dropping.

CATCH-UP SMOOTHIE

YIELD:
1 SMOOTHIE

PREP TIME:
5 MINUTES

COOK TIME:
0 MINUTES

Not every day will go perfectly according to your nutrition plan. I love this smoothie recipe for those days, because in just one drink you can cross a lot of items off your daily lower-cholesterol checklist. It has two servings of vegetables, two servings of fruit, a serving of nuts, and more than 100 percent of the daily recommended amount of alpha-linolenic acid (ALA), a form of omega-3s. You won't fall short with this catch-up smoothie.

1 celery stalk, roughly chopped

1 large carrot, roughly chopped

2 cups (60 g) fresh spinach or ½ cup (95 g) frozen spinach

1 tablespoon (15 ml) lemon or lime juice

1 teaspoon fresh or frozen ginger

½ apple, chopped

½ cup (80 g) frozen pineapple

2 tablespoons (15 g) walnuts

1 tablespoon (7 g) hemp seeds

2 cups (475 ml) water

Add all ingredients to a blender. Blend on high for 2 minutes or until all ingredients are thoroughly incorporated. Pour into a large glass or jar. Enjoy immediately or store in the refrigerator.

NUTRITIONAL ANALYSIS

SERVING SIZE: 1 smoothie

PER SERVING: 253 calories; 12 g fat; 1 g saturated fat; 8 g protein; 34 g carbohydrates; 8 g dietary fiber

HIGH-PROTEIN YOGURT BOWL

A high-protein yogurt bowl is the perfect snack when you are too hungry to make it to your next meal. With beneficial probiotics from the yogurt, antioxidants from the berries, omega-3s and healthy fats from the nuts, and a touch more protein from vanilla protein powder, this may become a staple of your afternoons.

■ YIELD:
1 SERVING

■ PREP TIME:
5 MINUTES

■ COOK TIME:
0 MINUTES

⅔ cup (153 g) 0 percent Greek yogurt

Vanilla protein powder, enough to add 10 g of protein

1 cup (155 g) fresh or frozen berries

1 tablespoon (8 g) walnuts

1 tablespoon (8 g) pistachios

Dash of cinnamon

Mix yogurt and protein powder vigorously in a bowl to thoroughly dissolve and combine protein powder. Top with berries, walnuts, pistachios, and cinnamon. Enjoy!

SUGGESTED COMBINATIONS AND TOPPINGS

Change up the combination of protein powder and toppings to customize this snack.

- Chocolate protein powder + 1 cup (78 g) frozen dark cherries + 2 tablespoons (16 g) pistachios

- Chocolate protein powder + 2 tablespoons (16 g) peanuts or peanut butter

- Vanilla protein powder + 1 cup (155 g) frozen pineapple + 2 tablespoons (16 g) crushed macadamia nuts

- Cinnamon protein powder + 2 tablespoons (20 g) pureed pumpkin + 2 tablespoons (20 g) pumpkin seeds

NUTRITIONAL ANALYSIS

SERVING SIZE: 1 yogurt bowl

PER SERVING: 293 calories; 8 g fat; 1 g saturated fat; 30 g protein; 28 g carbohydrates; 5 g dietary fiber

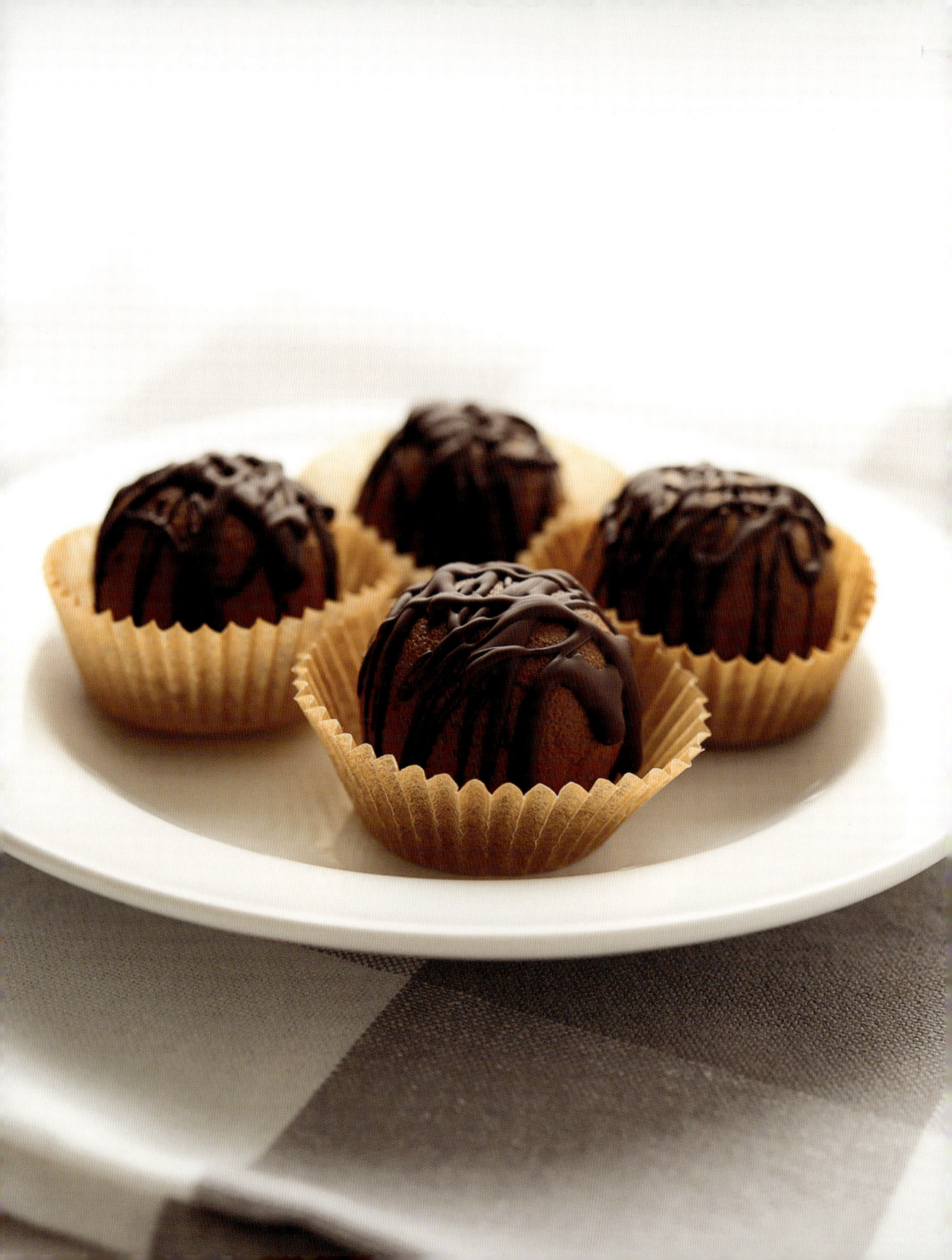

CHOCOLATE PEANUT BUTTER PROTEIN BALLS

■ **YIELD:**
1 SERVING

■ **PREP TIME:**
10 MINUTES

■ **COOK TIME:**
0 MINUTES

The protein in these balls comes entirely from peanut butter powder. Made from peanut butter with the fat removed, peanut butter powder retains a strong peanut flavor and protein. A lot of it, in fact! The pumpkin puree in this recipe acts as the binding agent and also provides some dietary fiber and beta-carotene, an important antioxidant. Drizzled with melted dark chocolate and spiced with cinnamon, these protein balls are a real heart-healthy treat.

¼ cup (65 g) peanut butter powder

¼ cup (61 g) pumpkin puree

1 tablespoon (5 g) cocoa powder

1 teaspoon maple syrup

¼ teaspoon pumpkin pie spice or cinnamon

1 tablespoon (11 g) dark chocolate chips

1 teaspoon milk

Mix peanut butter powder, pumpkin puree, cocoa powder, maple syrup, and spices together in a small bowl. Continue to stir until all ingredients are thoroughly combined and the color is dark brown. Roll the mixture into four 1-inch (2.5 cm) balls and place in the freezer for 5 minutes to harden.

In a separate microwave-safe bowl, add chocolate chips and milk. Microwave on high for 15 seconds at a time, stirring intermittently, until chocolate chips are completely melted and combined. Remove balls from the freezer. Drizzle with melted chocolate. Allow to cool for 1 to 2 minutes before eating.

These can be stored in the refrigerator for up to 1 week or frozen for up to 6 months.

NUTRITIONAL ANALYSIS

SERVING SIZE: 4 balls

PER SERVING: 230 calories; 8 g fat; 3 g saturated fat; 17 g protein; 27 g carbohydrates; 6 g dietary fiber

COTTAGE CHEESE DIP

This dip is incredibly simple, but it is an easy and versatile way to get in a high-protein snack that also provides some fiber. I highly recommend trying the other suggested sauces and seasonings in the Notes. Pair with high-fiber crackers and veggies, and enjoy!

■ **YIELD:**
1 SERVING

■ **PREP TIME:**
5 MINUTES

■ **COOK TIME:**
0 MINUTES

½ cup (115 g) low-fat cottage cheese

1 tablespoon (8 g) everything bagel seasoning

15 high-fiber crackers

6 carrot sticks

Add cottage cheese to a small bowl and top with everything bagel seasoning or a seasoning or sauce of your choice (see Suggested Toppings). Serve with crackers and carrots for dipping.

SUGGESTED TOPPINGS

You can top the cottage cheese with just about anything you like! Try these.

- 1 tablespoon (15 g) pesto
- 1 tablespoon (15 ml) Bitchin' Sauce
- 1 tablespoon (15 g) salsa
- 1 tablespoon (8 g) taco seasoning
- 1–2 teaspoons balsamic glaze

NUTRITIONAL ANALYSIS

SERVING SIZE: ½ cup (about 120 g) dip

PER SERVING: 330 calories; 8 g fat; 3 g saturated fat; 24 g protein; 27 g carbohydrates; 49 g dietary fiber

BEAN DIP WITH VEGGIES

Did you know you can make an easy bean dip at home from ingredients you already have sitting around in your pantry? While hummus is the most common bean dip, any type of bean will work in a creamy dip. It's a great option to keep stored in the refrigerator for curing snack-time hunger and helping to get in some extra fiber.

■ YIELD:
4 SERVINGS

■ PREP TIME:
10 MINUTES

■ COOK TIME:
0 MINUTES

1 (15.5-ounce [423 g]) can white or navy beans, drained and rinsed

2 garlic cloves, chopped

1 tablespoon (15 ml) water

1 teaspoon lemon juice

1 tablespoon (15 ml) olive oil

¼ teaspoon salt

½ teaspoon ground cumin

4 carrots, cut into sticks

6 celery stalks, cut into sticks

1 medium cucumber, sliced

1 cup (150 g) cherry tomatoes

Add beans, garlic, and water to a food processor. Process until beans form a smooth and creamy paste, about 60 seconds. Add lemon juice, olive oil, salt, and cumin. Process for another 30 seconds. Serve in a ramekin with fresh vegetables for dipping.

Store in an airtight container in the refrigerator for up to 1 week.

NUTRITIONAL ANALYSIS

SERVING SIZE: ¼ cup (about 80 g) bean dip + 1 cup (130 g) veggies

PER SERVING: 189 calories; 1 g fat; 0 g saturated fat; 10 g protein; 38 g carbohydrates; 10 g dietary fiber

EDAMAME CORN SALAD

A tangy and flavorful salad filled with plant-based protein and a hefty amount of fiber for a snack, this edamame corn salad is a great option to store in the fridge for when you need a snack that will help keep you full for a few hours. Plus, most of these ingredients are shelf stable, so this can be whipped up at any time.

YIELD:
1 SERVING

PREP TIME:
10 MINUTES

COOK TIME:
0 MINUTES

¾ cup (128 g) frozen edamame

½ cup (65 g) frozen corn

1 green onion, both green and white parts, thinly sliced

¼ cup (38 g) cherry tomatoes, halved or quartered

1 teaspoon pesto

1 teaspoon red wine vinegar

1 tablespoon (9 g) feta cheese

Add frozen edamame and corn to a medium bowl. Cover with hot water for 4 to 5 minutes, or until the edamame and corn have thawed.

Once thawed, drain water and dump the vegetables onto a paper towel to dry. Add them and the remaining ingredients to a bowl. Toss to coat everything in the pesto and vinegar. Enjoy!

NUTRITIONAL ANALYSIS

SERVING SIZE: 1½ cups
(about 240 g) salad

PER SERVING: 289 calories; 10 g fat; 2 g saturated fat; 18 g protein; 33 g carbohydrates; 9 g dietary fiber

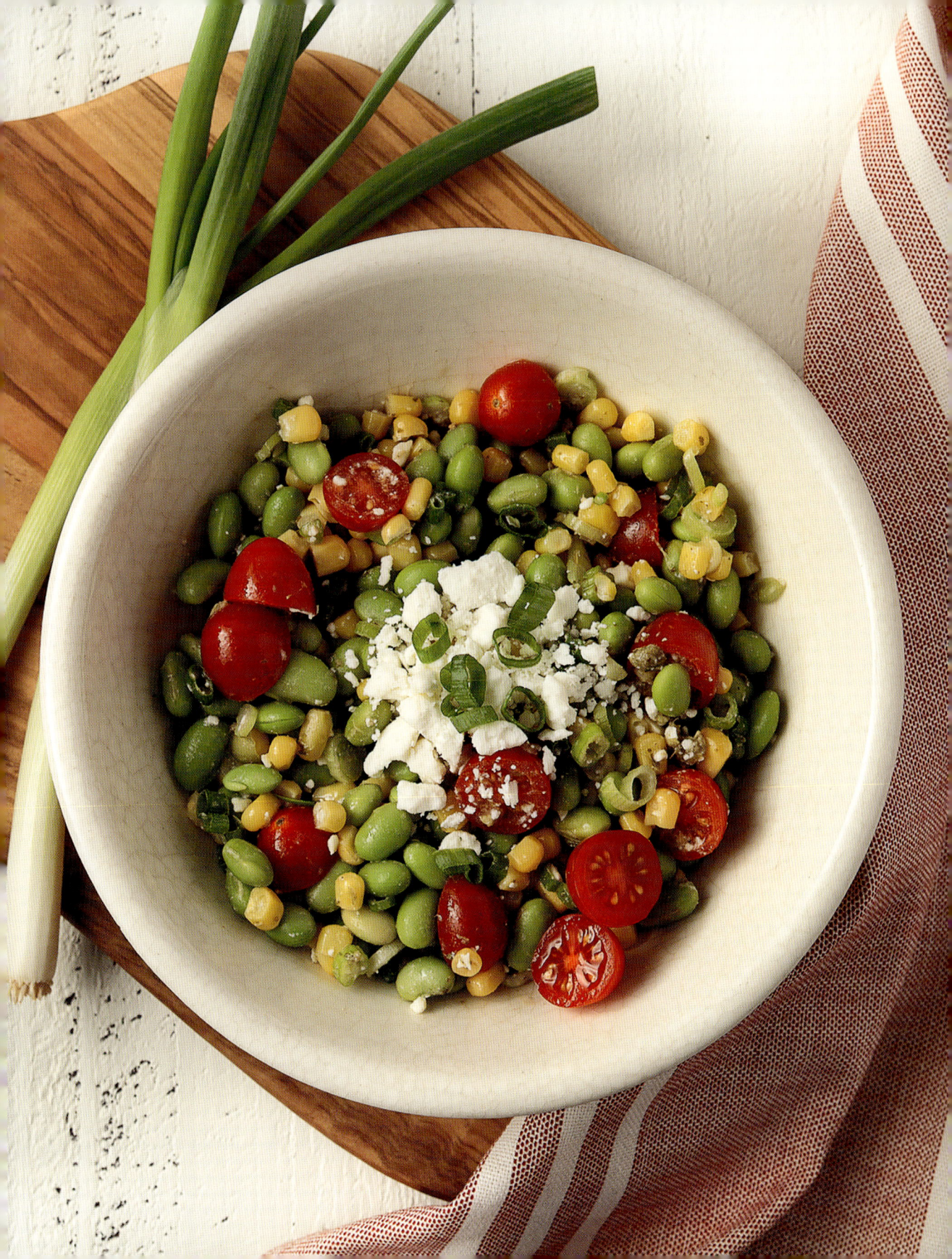

LOW-CHOLESTEROL ADULT LUNCH-ABLE

■ **YIELD:**
1 SERVING

■ **PREP TIME:**
5 MINUTES

■ **COOK TIME:**
5 MINUTES

A snack box is not just for kids. It works for adults too. If you were a kid or had a kid in the 90s, you likely remember Lunchables. They were fun to eat because they came in their own compartmentalized container and offered a lot of variety. The concept works great for packing snacks too. This "lunch-able" has a balance of protein, fat, carbs, and fiber to give y ou a pick-me-up when you need a snack.

- 1 tablespoon (9 g) dry roasted peanuts
- 2 tablespoons (21 g) dried edamame
- 1 low-fat mozzarella string cheese
- 2 prunes
- 4 woven wheat crackers, like Triscuits

Using a four-compartment container, organize your ingredients into sections. Mix together peanuts and edamame in one compartment. Slice string cheese into 4 bite-size pieces for another. Cut prunes into quarters to make them bite-size and place in their own compartment. Add crackers to the final compartment. Cover with a lid to keep fresh and make portable. Eat directly from the container. Pairing the cheese, prunes, and crackers in one bite is a delicious way to enjoy this box. Or eat each compartment by itself—whatever sounds most appealing to you.

SUGGESTED COMBINATIONS

There are endless possibilities for this adult lunch-able. Be mindful of the total saturated fat in your lunch-able and make sure to include some high-fiber and high-protein items!

- Mini cheese, like Babybel
- Greek yogurt mixed with ranch powder to create a ranch-style dip
- Cottage cheese topped with everything bagel seasoning
- Two dates filled with peanut butter
- Edamame in the pod
- Seed-based crackers (I like Mary's Gone Crackers)
- Chocolate Peanut Butter Protein Ball (page 145)

NUTRITIONAL ANALYSIS

SERVING SIZE: 1 lunch-able

PER SERVING: 292 calories; 12 g fat; 4 g saturated fat; 16 g protein; 29 g carbohydrates; 6 g dietary fiber

CHEESECAKE DIP WITH FRESH STRAWBERRIES

■ **YIELD:**
1 SERVING

■ **PREP TIME:**
5 MINUTES

■ **COOK TIME:**
0 MINUTES

Another winner in the cottage cheese book is this cheesecake dip. It's delicious when served with fresh fruit and provides a healthy dose of protein to help you arrive at your next meal hungry but not starving!

⅔ cup (150 g) low-fat cottage cheese

Vanilla protein powder, enough to add 10 g of protein

2 cups (290 g) fresh strawberries, halved or quartered

Using a food processor or immersion blender, blend cottage cheese and protein powder until it reaches a smooth and creamy consistency. Serve with fresh strawberries for dipping.

NUTRITIONAL ANALYSIS

SERVING SIZE: ⅔ cup (about 150 g) dip + 2 cups (290 g) strawberries

PER SERVING: 275 calories; 1 g fat; 3 g saturated fat; 30 g protein; 40 g carbohydrates; 8 g dietary fiber

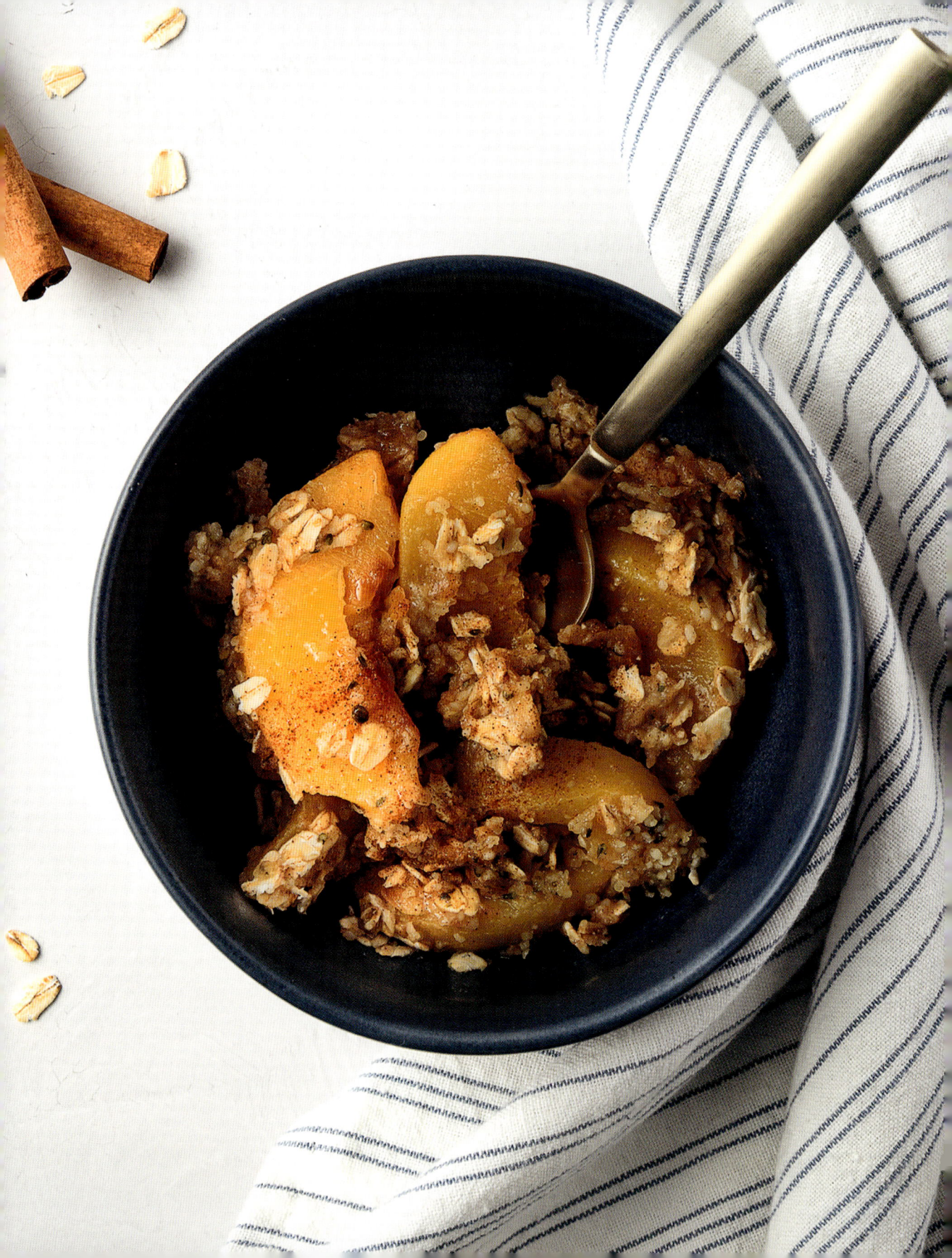

MICROWAVE PEACH COBBLER

When the need for a sweet treat strikes, this microwave cobbler absolutely hits the spot! Made with frozen fruit, it never goes out of season. Just be sure to let it cool for a few minutes before enjoying so you don't burn your mouth!

YIELD:
1 SERVING

PREP TIME:
5 MINUTES

COOK TIME:
5 MINUTES

FOR THE COBBLER

1 cup (250 g) frozen peaches

⅛ teaspoon cinnamon

1½ teaspoons flour

1 tablespoon (15 ml) water

FOR THE CRUMBLE TOPPING

2 tablespoons (10 g) rolled oats

1 tablespoon (8 g) flour

1½ teaspoons brown sugar

⅛ teaspoon salt

1 tablespoon (7 g) hemp seeds

1½ teaspoons plant-based butter, cold, finely diced or shredded

⅛ teaspoon cinnamon

TO MAKE THE COBBLER

Add fruit to a microwave-safe dish with cinnamon. Microwave for 90 seconds on high or until fruit is bubbly and hot. Remove from microwave and add flour and water, stirring thoroughly to combine. Set aside.

TO MAKE THE CRUMBLE TOPPING

Next, mix together the crumble topping ingredients in a separate bowl. Use your fingers to break up the butter and incorporate throughout the mixture.

Evenly distribute crumble on top of fruit and flour mixture. Microwave for 2 minutes. Give the dish a stir to incorporate the fruit juices with the crumble topping. Allow cobbler to sit for 3 to 4 minutes after cooking to cool before enjoying.

NOTES

- To make with berries, substitute 1½ teaspoons lemon juice for water.

- To make with fresh apple: Core and dice 1 apple and microwave for 2 minutes instead of 90 seconds. Add ⅛ teaspoon each of nutmeg and ground clove too.

NUTRITIONAL ANALYSIS

SERVING SIZE: 1 cobbler

PER SERVING: 273 calories; 11 g fat; 2 g saturated fat; 7 g protein; 38 g carbohydrates; 4 g dietary fiber

CHOCOLATE "CHICK" COOKIE DOUGH

■ YIELD:
8 SERVINGS

■ PREP TIME:
10 MINUTES

■ COOK TIME:
0 MINUTES

Go ahead, get a spoon! Made without egg or flour, this cookie dough made from chickpeas (hence the name), peanut butter, and maple syrup is 100 percent safe to eat "raw" and right from the container. And it still makes great cookies when baked!

1 cup (175 g) prunes

¼ cup (60 ml) boiling water

1 (15.5-ounce [423 g]) can no-salt-added chickpeas, drained and rinsed

⅓ cup (27 g) rolled oats

⅓ cup (86 g) peanut butter

¼ cup (80 g) maple syrup

2 teaspoons vanilla extract

½ teaspoon cinnamon

⅛ teaspoon salt

Room temperature water, as needed

⅓ cup (58 g) dark chocolate chips

Add prunes to a small bowl and carefully cover in boiling water to soak for about 5 minutes.

Add chickpeas, oats, peanut butter, maple syrup, vanilla extract, cinnamon, and salt to a food processor. When the prunes are done soaking, add the prunes and the water to the processor as well. Blend on high for 3 to 4 minutes. If your dough looks too thick, add 1 tablespoon (15 ml) water while the processor is running. Continue to add 1 tablespoon (15 ml) water at a time until you reach your desired consistency. Stir in chocolate chips.

You can eat this chocolate chip cookie dough straight from the container with a spoon because there are no raw eggs or flour that needs to be cooked. It can also serve as a dip for apples or strawberries, rolled into balls and frozen for 5 to 10 minutes, or baked into cookies (see Note).

NUTRITIONAL ANALYSIS

SERVING SIZE: 2 tablespoons (about 115 g) dough

PER SERVING: 228 calories; 9 g fat; 2 g saturated fat; 5 g protein; 33 g carbohydrates; 4 g dietary fiber

NOTE

To make these into egg- and gluten-free chocolate chip cookies, use a spoon or scoop to drop tablespoons of the dough onto a baking sheet lined with parchment paper and sprayed with nonstick spray. Bake for 10 minutes at 350°F (180°C or gas mark 4).

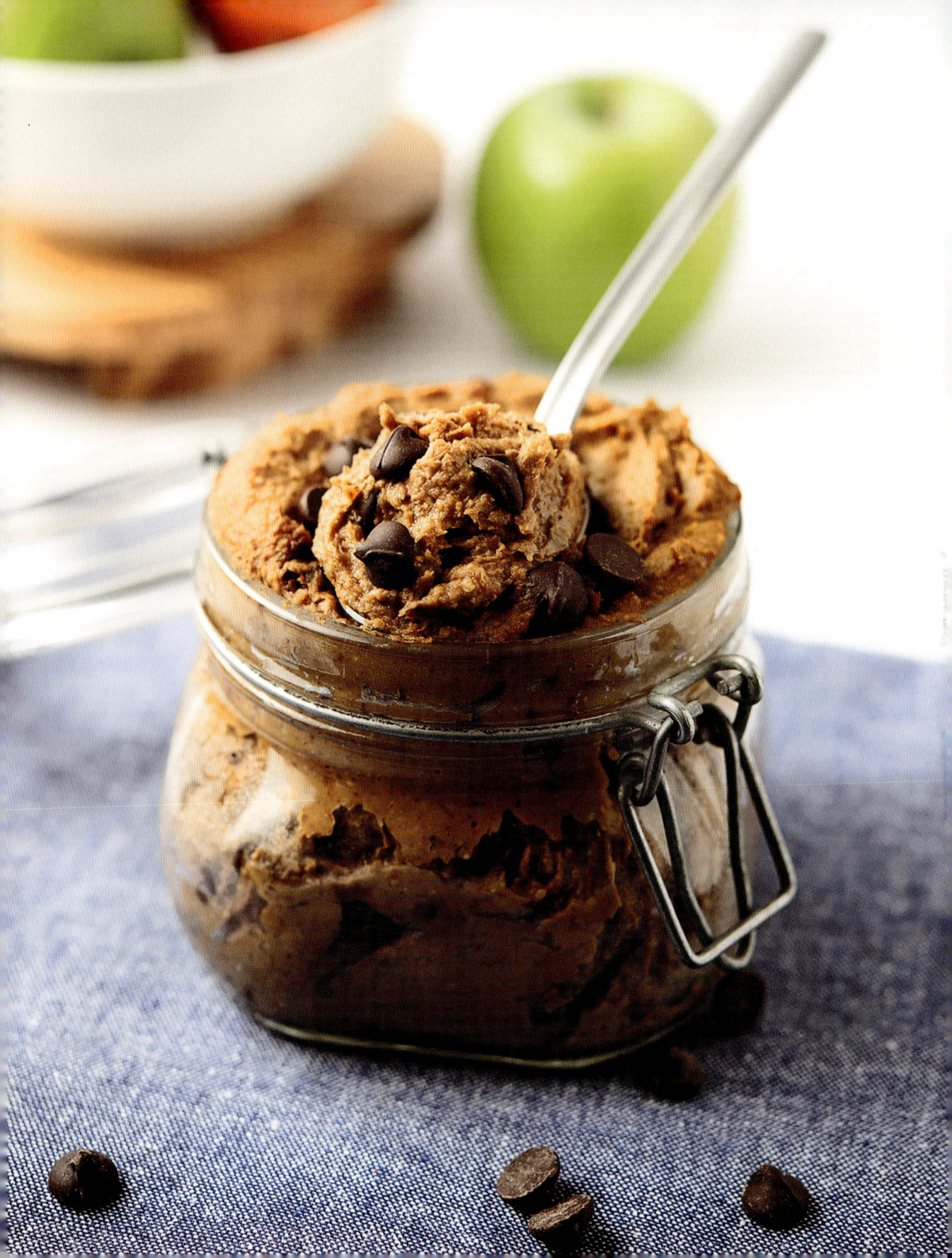

References

CHAPTER 1

American Heart Association. "Life's Essential 8." Heart.org. https://www.heart.org/en/healthy-living/healthy-lifestyle/lifes-essential-8.

Cockerill G, and Xu Q. "Atherosclerosis." *Mechanisms of Vascular Disease: A Reference Book for Vascular Specialists*, edited by Robert Fitridge and Matthew Thompson. University of Adelaide Press, 2011: pp. 3.

National Lipid Association. (n.d.). *CLM Training and Resources*, https://www.lipid.org/clmt.

Thomas DT, et al. "Position of the Academy of Nutrition and Dietetics, Dietitians of Canada, and the American College of Sports Medicine: Nutrition and Athletic Performance." *J Acad Nutr Diet.* 2016; 116,3: 501–528. doi.org/10.1016/j.jand.2015.12.006.

Tsao CW, Aday AW, Almarzooq ZI, Beaton AZ, Bittencourt MS, Boehme AK, et al. "Heart Disease and Stroke Statistics—2023 Update: A Report from the American Heart Association." *Circulation.* 2023;147:e93–e621. doi.org/10.1161/cir.0000000000001123.

U.S. Department of Agriculture and U.S. Department of Health and Human Services. *Dietary Guidelines for Americans, 2020-2025*, 9th edition. December 2020. http://www.dietaryguidelines.gov/resources/2020-2025-dietary-guidelines-online-materials.

United States Department of Agriculture. *FoodData Central.* U.S. Department of Agriculture. https://fdc.nal.usda.gov.

Resources

American Heart Association, heart.org

Hachfeld, Linda, and Amy Myrdal Miller. *Cooking à la Heart: 500 Easy and Delicious Recipes for Heart-Conscious, Healthy Meals*, 4th edition. Foreword by James M. Rippe. Workman Publishing, 2023.

Lower Cholesterol, Longer Life Method. This self-paced course is available at www.ashleyreaver.com.

National Lipid Association, nla.org

Acknowledgments

This cookbook would not have been possible without the support, inspiration, and contributions of many incredible people.

To my mom and dad, thanks for the unending love and support, encouragement in cooking from a young age, and the push to branch out on my own path as a dietitian.

To my husband, Eric, for rarely complaining about food and for being the first to test (and sometimes endure!) my cooking experiments.

To my son, Miles, for making me want to put healthy meals on the table each day and explore how fun food can be.

To my friends, thank you for sharing my love of food and always being open to sharing a good meal.

A heartfelt thanks to Hilary Vandenbroek and the team at Quarto, whose expertise and creativity transformed my vision into reality. Your dedication and talent shine through every page.

To my mentors and colleagues who have supported my passion for food and nutrition over the years. Every person has taught me valuable lessons that have shaped me into the person and dietitian I am today.

To my culinary inspirations, whether through books, shows, or personal lessons, your guidance has profoundly influenced my cooking journey. A special shoutout to the Food Network 3 to 6 p.m. time slot in 2004 for first inspiring my love of cooking.

Finally, to you, the reader—thank you for bringing this book into your kitchen. May it inspire delicious meals, remove stress from the eating process, and lower your cholesterol levels.

About the Author

Ashley Reaver is a registered dietitian and certified specialist in sports dietetics. She received her undergraduate degree in nutrition sciences and dietetics from Cornell University and a master's in nutrition science and policy from Tufts University. She is a full-time lecturer in nutritional sciences and dietetics at the University of California, Berkeley, and owns a private nutrition practice, Ashley Reaver Nutrition. Her previous experience as a dietitian includes food service management, personalized health analytics, and corporate wellness. Her private practice focuses on cardiovascular health, specifically cholesterol. She is the coauthor of *The Postpartum Nutrition Cookbook*, a resource for healing from pregnancy and birth. She lives in California with her husband, Eric, and son, Miles. She is an avid hiker, home cook, and gardener. Follow her on Instagram @lower.cholesterol.nutrition.

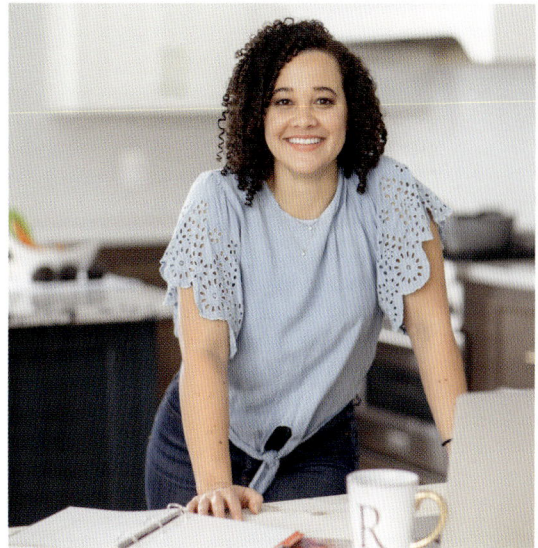

Index